Shiatsu

Space for Encounter

Edited by

Barbara Murakami

Pirmoni Verlag

www.pirmoni.de

Bibliografische Information der Deutschen Nationalbibliothek:
Die Deutsche Nationalbibliothek verzeichnet diese Publikation in der Deutschen Nationalbibliografie; detaillierte bibliografische Daten sind im Internet über www.dnb.dnb.de abrufbar.

Picture credits:
pp. 7,29,33,45,67, 89,99,109,121,145,161,203 © Pirmoni-Verlag, Krefeld
p. 79 © taken from the Daoist canon, 13 Jh., »Gebieter der vier Richtungen«
p.133 © with friendly permission of Ulrike Haffke
p. 153 © with friendly permission of Susanne Jüsten
p. 179 © Cave painting based on the *Cueva de las manos*
p. 187 © Angelika Bungert-Stüttgen, www.freiraumfrau.de
The copyright of the portrait photos in the appendix lies with the respective authors.

Cover design:
Im Bambushain, Krefeld, Germany

Printed by:
TOTEM, Polen

ISBN 978-3-9825990-2-1 (Paperback)
ISBN 978-3-9825990-3-8 (ebook)

Contents

Foreword 5

1 Finding Authentic Connection 7
Barbara Murakami

2 DJ 27
Heidy van Koesveld

3 Being in Suspension 31
Rami Leon Yulzari

4 From Practitioner to Companion 41
Joachim Schrievers

5 Pictures in a Treatment Room 61
Rami Leon Yulzari

6 The Alchemy of Words 71
Chris McAlister

7 To Speak or Not to Speak? 81
Chris McAlister

8 Zen, Shiatsu and the Art of the Clown 89
Nick Pole

9 Muscles have Feelings Too 97
Bill Palmer

10 Like a Caterpillar in a Cocoon 107
Barbara Murakami

11 The Spirit of the Curtain 119
Rami Leon Yulzari

12 Resonance in Body Therapy 129
Wilfried Rappenecker

13 Images of Resonance 135
Rami Leon Yulzari

14 The Transpersonal Field of Experience as a Resonance Phenomenon 143
Joachim Schrievers

15 Human Dignity is Tangible 159
René Fix

16 Sound of the Heart, NOW 167
Rami Leon Yulzari

17 Walking to talk 181
Chris McAlister

Authors 187

Foreword

As the editor, co-author and translator of this book, »Shiatsu – Space for Encounter,« it is a pleasure for me to preface its English edition with a few introductory words. Within these pages, you will find a narrative that transcends the mere mechanics of Shiatsu practice, delving into the essence of what it means to truly connect with another human being.

In reflecting on the essence of Shiatsu, I am reminded of a poignant conversation with my dear friend and mentor, Joachim Schrievers. Over pizza and red wine, he posed a simple yet profound question: »What is the core of Shiatsu?« After a moment of silence, my answer emerged effortlessly: »To be with someone for a while.« Was that a suitable answer? I don't think you would find it on the website of a Shiatsu practitioner. Yet, while seemingly simplistic and vague, this notion seemed to encapsulate the heart of Shiatsu – a practice rooted not only in technique, but in the genuine presence and connection between practitioner and recipient.

After a thorough training in the theoretical basics and all those various treatment techniques of Shiatsu, my journey into the heart of Shiatsu began through my regular work with severely disabled adults.

At first, I was at a loss. Most of what I had learned so far was unsuitable for this situation. People who have been sitting in a wheelchair almost motionless for most of their lives don't care about meridians, skillful stretches or rotations. And even those who can walk or even lie down on the mat can often do little with a »classic« shiatsu treatment or initially find it very difficult to engage with touch.

It would have stood to reason to throw in the towel with the understanding that Shiatsu made no sense in this context. Something stopped me, however, and every week I patiently invited the people entrusted to me to spend time with »Shiatsu«.

The miracle happened in slow motion. Over a period of months tender threads of contact were spun and gradually developed into stable, cordial connections. Many of my clients were increasingly happy to accept my offer, they put my hands to where they wanted to be touched and moved in a shared rhythm with me, we just enjoyed times of silence and we always found a way to a smile or a hearty laugh. These encounters touched me deeply and made it even clearer to me than I had already known from my own previous experiences with Shiatsu: I discovered that the true magic of Shiatsu lies in the quiet moments of shared presence and connection. The core of Shiatsu is encounter, is authentic connection. Could this also be an answer to the initial question?

I immersed myself in this exploration and, as Milton Erickson, the founder of hypnotherapy says: »Energy flows, where the attention goes.« That's, what happened. I found myself surrounded by a community of fellow practitioners who shared their own insights and experiences on the subject of encounter in Shiatsu. That's how the idea for this book came about. It is intended to bundle the widely scattered experiences and insights like a magnifying glass and to draw the eye onto the core of Shiatsu, to connection, to encounter, to what happens between the two partners in the process. By shining a light on the subtle dynamics that unfold between practitioner and recipient, we can uncover a deeper understanding of the healing potential inherent in these connections.

It is with sincere gratitude that I extend my heartfelt thanks to all the wonderful colleagues who have contributed to this book. Their expertise, wisdom, support and generosity have been invaluable in bringing this project to fruition. This book would not have been possible without their contributions.

And I would like to sincerely thank Nick Pole, Chris McAllister, Heidy van Koesveld, and Garry Hammond for their invaluable assistance in refining the translations contained within this book. Their expertise and attention to detail have helped to ensure that the essence of these teachings remains true to the original intent.

With each word carefully translated, my hope is that the essence of Shiatsu – rooted in the power of authentic connection – will resonate with readers from diverse cultures and backgrounds. It is my belief that the universal language of touch and human connection knows no bounds, transcending geographical borders and linguistic barriers.

»I wish there had been a book like this during my Shiatsu training«, someone said to whom I gave these texts to read in advance.

Well, here it is and I hope you enjoy reading it.

Barbara Murakami, April 2024

1

Barbara Murakami

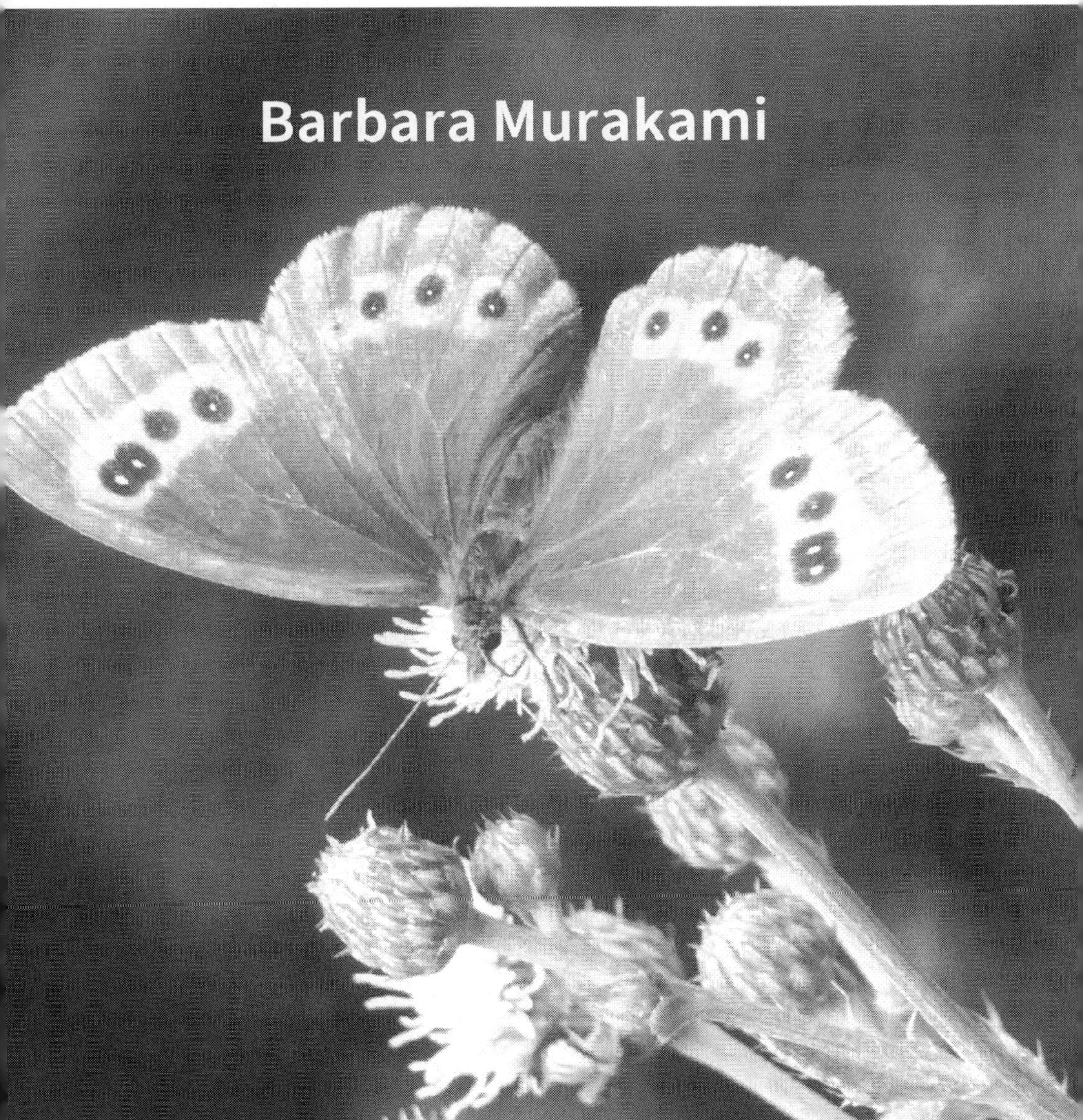

Finding Authentic Connection

BUILDING RELATIONSHIPS IN SHIATSU

”

**He who marvels
cannot at the same time
reject or devalue.**

Lukas

»Leave again«, says Lukas, an autistic young man, after the first two minutes of his Shiatsu treatment. Lukas is 29 years old, tall and thin with large, absent eyes and hasty movements. Eye contact is almost impossible. He speaks very little and then in short, choppy sentences. He wears his headphones. He always carries them with him, along with his MP3 player. He is a new member of the group of adults in an institution for people with disabilities who receive Shiatsu from me on a regular basis as part of a personal development programme.

So we go back to his workplace. The following week I pick him up again, take him to the room I can use for the treatments, he sits down on the bench (he doesn't lie down, certainly not on a mat on the floor), I treat his hands. After three minutes, at his request, I take him back.

Over the next few weeks, our meetings follow a similar pattern. I pick him up, he lets me treat him for a few minutes and then he wants to go back to his workplace. However, a slow – motion development is taking place, which becomes clear when you look back six months later.

Now, when I stand in the doorway to pick him up, he immediately runs across the room to take my hand, smiles, and quickly walks off with me. He has a name for what it's all about: »Shiatsu«. He has been asking about it all morning. In the treatment room, he immediately sits down on the bench and holds out his hands to me. We always start the treatment with his hands. His eyes wander around the room and he asks me to put things in order, like closing the door to an adjoining room or turning the light on or off. Of course, I comply. I work on his arms, shoulders, back and legs as he sits. Every now and then he makes eye contact with me and we smile at each other. It now takes 15 minutes or more before he wants to leave again. When I meet him in the corridor later that day, he says: »The Shiatsu was good«.

»Finding Authentic Connection« is the title of this essay. The brief description of a series of treatments with an autistic person illustrates some of the conditions for fruitful contact in Shiatsu, as it is more difficult for autistic people to make contact at all than for others.

- An authentic connection is only possible when the client can fully trust that nothing will happen that is contrary to their needs, that they are in control of the situation and that there is no imbalance of power. Only then can they can engage and open up.

- At the same time, it is about actively responding to the client's needs. Would they prefer to sit, lie or stand? Which areas of the body need touch? (Some of the disabled people I work with may not be able to speak, but they guide my hands to where they want to be touched). Should the heating or lights be on or off?

- A relationship is most easily established when two people are »on the same wavelength« in at least one area. In the context of Shiatsu, this means that the practitioner first tunes into the energy of the person being treated in a mutual resonance. This tuning can manifest itself in the practitioner adjusting the speed at which they move and speak to match that of the client, using a similar volume, adopting a similar posture and also adjusting their facial expressions to match the client's. In psychotherapy this is called pacing. In the language of Traditional Chinese Medicine, it is about a yin quality in the treatment, as well as the point of »responding to the client's needs«. In the case of Lukas, for example, this means going along with his erratic movements rather than counteracting them and to some extent picking up on his short, choppy sentences.

- Encounters need a counterpart. What I have said about pacing does not mean that the practitioner should withdraw completely. It is only when they show themselves with their own joy, dismay or vulnerability, when they bring impulses into the process of their own accord that trigger development, when they also set limits to the client's needs, that a real contact can arise. In psychotherapy, this is known as leading; in the language of TCM, it is known as a yang quality.

- It often takes a lot of patience to create space for encounter and development. It might have been tempting to stop Lukas' treatments after 2-3 attempts with the thought: Shiatsu is not for him. But then this fulfilling development would not have taken place. »Grass does not grow faster if you pull on it« is an African proverb. This is also true for Shiatsu. You can create the space for growth, but the growth itself must happen at its own pace.

- Perseverance and repetition are closely linked to patience. Deep encounters and sustainable development usually require more than just a single event.

Inner Practice – It's all a Matter of Attitude

Let us now leave the realm of this particular form of Shiatsu treatment for a while and turn our attention to the subject of attitudes. To answer this question, we will turn to psychology and philosophy, among other things, because encounter is also a psychological process.

What exactly is encounter?

Today, instead of connection or encounter, we often come across the term resonance. The sociologist Hartmut Rosa has studied resonance extensively and has identified four characteristics:

- **Touch:** When I resonate with someone, they touch me inside, something in my soul is set in motion, attention and interest are aroused, my eyes widen or begin to light up.

- **Self-efficacy:** However, I can only speak of resonance when I enter into an exchange with the other person and reach them. Glances are exchanged, a physical reaction may become visible, a dialogue develops on a physical or verbal level.

- **Transformation:** Through the experience of resonance, something changes in me and in the other person. This can be something big, something that »makes me into a different person« or something barely perceptible such as a temporary change in mood or view of something.

- **Uncontrollability:** Whether or not resonance occurs is beyond our control. Although we can create some conditions that favour resonance, we cannot force it. Nor do we really have any real influence on the direction in which a change moves and what the result will be. We will come back to this point at a later stage.

Immediacy

At the beginning of a Shiatsu treatment, as many of us have learned during our training, there is usually a diagnosis, which is differentiated and changed during the course of the treatment. This may be a hara diagnosis, a questioning, a pulse diagnosis or an examination of the whole energy field. After the treatment, we often take some notes to use as a basis for further treatments.

I still remember my own training days. One of our homework assignments was to write reports on several series of 10 treatments. What struck me immediately was the fact that what happens in the depths of Shiatsu is not really something that can be put into words. So, everything I put down on paper just stayed on the surface. And taking notes had the effect of focusing my attention more on the describable surface phenomena, so that I could find something that could be categorised as a concept and written down. It was easy to lose sight of the person as a whole with his or her developmental tasks and possibilities. The woman lying in front of me then became the one with the helper syndrome and the Kyo in the spleen meridian, another one became the woman with depression and neediness in the metal area.

I also remember the treatments I received myself at the time. How many times did I try to understand from a theoretical point of view what the practitioner was doing? Which meridian had he chosen? What techniques did he use? What did the Hara diagnosis reveal?

This resulted in me not being fully engaged in the actual process, but rather perceiving what the meridian concepts suggested was happening.

Diagnoses and protocols are important to give direction to what we do. But they get in the way of a real encounter in the present moment. An encounter is immediate. Neither previous experiences nor concepts, expectations and desires come between the two people who meet. »No memory, no desire, no understanding!« is also the advice of the psychoanalyst Wilfred Bion in relation to psychotherapeutic processes, because according to him, memories, desires and explanations prevent intuition and receptivity to what is really happening in the moment, to the ultimate truth shared by the two people meeting.

The religious philosopher Martin Buber distinguishes between two basic attitudes from which a person can relate to the world. From the attitude of I-It, I perceive the world in detail, interpret it, make it available, shape it. I stand in front of a something or even several somethings that are separated from me and from each other. From the attitude of I-Thou, I grasp the other person with my whole being in their entirety. I do not perceive them as a thing, and they are not made up of things. This is Buber's analogy to illustrate the point:

»Just as the melody is not made up of notes, nor a verse is of words … so is the man to whom I say Thou. I can take out from him the colour of his hair, or of his speech or of his goodness, I must continually do this. But each time I do it he ceases to be Thou.«

Children in particular are able to observe the other in a holistic, self-forgetting way. They can stand in front of a person with their mouth open, their eyes wide, without any reaction of their own and take them in completely. This kind of observation is what we call »marvelling«. It shows great respect and refrains from any judgement.

»He who marvels cannot at the same time reject or devalue«, writes Mechthild Erpenbeck in her book *Wirksam werden im Kontakt.* »It is not even possible to explain and to understand. In moments of pure marvelling, we are literally speechless and self-forgetful. This can be a very valuable foundation for all subsequent actions in our work: Once the moment of wonder has passed, a curious, cautious movement towards it follows. Just like the toddler in the underground who, after long minutes of silent wonder, ›awakens‹ from his motionlessness and reaches out, for example, to the dreadlocks of the person sitting opposite to him. A cautious and yet determined gesture. It is the beginning of all that is meant by the word ›encounter‹. All exploration begins with this primal scene of marvelling. All use of knowledge and skill comes afterwards.«

This already suggests that it is neither possible nor sensible to approach the world from an I-Thou attitude throughout. The moment of wonder is just as fleeting as the moments of deep encounter. Consciousness soon swings back to an I-It attitude, and that is a good thing.

For we can only shape the world if we perceive it in detail and organise our perceptions into hypotheses, theories and concepts. Otherwise, we could neither communicate nor cooperate, let alone act and survive as individuals or as a community.

And of course, in Shiatsu, we need knowledge, techniques, and good diagnostics to support our clients with their particular problems.

What is important is the ability to oscillate between an openness and receptivity beyond all concepts, memories and expectations and a rational, deductive, evaluative and proactive attitude.

And so, perhaps unlike Bion, I would also see understanding as an important part of the therapeutic process. But it is only after the holistic encounter and perception that it has its place as an anchor for memory, as a guide for further work. Knowing full well that what I think I have understood is not permanent. If it becomes too prominent in our consciousness, it obscures our view of what may have already changed.

As important as it is to acquire knowledge, make diagnoses and pursue hypotheses, it is just as important to keep the windshield wipers on, to forget all previous knowledge and to be open to all the possibilities that the present moment holds. The Zen Buddhist Shunryu Suzuku coined the apt term »beginner‘s mind« for this, writing:

> »In the beginner's mind there are many possibilities, in the expert's mind there are only a few.«

A Soft Gaze

Time and space often fade into the background of my consciousness when I give Shiatsu. My brain is in alpha mode, as neurophysiologists call this state of heightened perceptual awareness of a wider field of internal and external processes, a state between waking and dream. I usually start by asking what theme the client has brought with them. This theme will then resonate and give a certain colour to the field without becoming too sharply defined.

A receptivity to what is unfolding right now is best established when our attention is not focused on specific objects, details or points, but is allowed to move freely in space. Free-floating attention is therefore also an attitude that is often adopted in psychotherapy in order to gain a sense of the current mental process as a whole. This type of attention allows everything that comes into awareness to stand side by side on an equal footing, without classifying, evaluating or weighting it. In psychoanalysis, it is therefore also called »evenly suspended attention«.

»Free-floating attention« does not mean that I can freely indulge in my thoughts and arbitrarily direct my attention to anything that comes to mind. That would be inattention.

The focus is on full attention to the process as a whole, with everything that arises in connection with the client and the practitioner. This need not be something outwardly perceptible such as a movement or an expression. In Shiatsu in particular, we work with the much more subtle perceptible movements of Qi, in the client, in the practitioner and in the whole energetic field. These can be perceptions that cannot yet be put into words and perhaps only take shape in inner images and daydreams.

Many of us are probably familiar with daydream-like states from Shiatsu treatments, whether in the role of the practitioner or the client. Giving them space can be a wonderful way to bring the energetic, unconscious processes of both participants into resonance. The psychoanalyst Bion calls this state of 'dreaming along' Rêverie, which the therapist can consciously adopt. What a poetic expression!

When two people meet in such a space of gentle attention, as Rami Yulzari, Shiatsu and Qigong teacher from Israel, calls it in his essay »Being in Suspension«, it is much easier to open up and make deep contact, because no one has to fear being prematurely categorised and judged. They can show themselves as they really are.

Being in Agreement

I've never had good posture. »Child, sit up straight«, my mother admonished me again and again, with the result that, in defiance, I slouched even more. A lot of desk work and the burden of everyday life did their bit. My upper back is not really straight like a dancer's and tends to be rather stiff. One of my first Shiatsu therapists meant well with me. He remarked that my upper back was very tense. With enthusiasm, he launched into the treatment, applying strong, rhythmic pressure to my thoracic spine. It was presumably intended for relaxation. Everything inside me tightened. My back tensed strongly to build up counter-pressure. »Leave me alone!« was my greatest wish in this situation.

In my opinion, being able to show yourself and being acknowledged unconditionally are basic prerequisites for contact. And it is from this point that further development is possible. Even if we like to fight against all sorts of things and want to change them, experience shows that things can only start to flow when we see and appreciate what we find for what it is. Yes, that's how it is … In Shiatsu, for example, this means that we are better off not offering hasty solutions to what we see as the client's problem. There are several reasons for this:

- The client gets the feeling that something is wrong with them. They will cut off the contact.

- The solution may not fit the nature or size of the problem. The client feels that their suffering and their own attempts to solve the problem are not seen and withdraws.

- A real solution to the problem will be more sustainable if the client finds it themselves, perhaps with our support. This can happen in conversation, but also by experimenting with different movements and touches.

- Perhaps what appears to us as the problem is a solution to something deeper that makes sense for the client. The first step is to recognise this. What does this ›problem‹ make possible for me? What does it prevent me from? What does it protect me from? (the stiff neck, the aching knee, the drug addiction …). These can be helpful questions that acknowledge what exists and at the same time initiate a reorientation.

- Recognising something as a fact can bring relaxation and peace even in very stressful situations. Yes, that's right, my back hurts. Yes, that's right, this important project failed. Yes, that's right, my life is coming to an end … Yes, that's how it is, and where can it go from here?

About Authorities, Experts and Eye Level

»My doctor diagnosed me with Restless Legs Syndrome. Can you do anything about it?« This was the inquiry from an elderly lady on the phone. »I can't sleep at all, and neither can my husband.« I listened to the lady for a while. My sympathy grew and so did my desire to help her. Nevertheless, I made an effort not to let her role ascription snap into place. »There's probably not much I can do on my own«, was my reply. »Let's see what we can achieve together.«

People often come to a Shiatsu treatment with a specific problem that the expert (practitioner) is supposed to fix. The practitioner as an authority. This is often the initial situation that needs to be acknowledged first. »Recognising what is.«

Indeed, Shiatsu practitioners usually undergo several years of training, acquiring extensive knowledge about meridian pathways and energetic connections. They have worked intensively on their inner attitude and outer posture and have learned many techniques.

They have acquired expertise and thus an authority in their field, which they provide to the client with the hope that it will improve their well-being soon. What could be wrong with that? Nothing at all for a start.

When it comes to financial matters, I turn to the tax advisor. If my car has an engine problem, the car mechanic is the expert, and I grant them a certain authority.

What about Shiatsu? In my opinion, it depends on three things: the degree of neediness of the client, the degree of personal responsibility that the client is currently willing and able to assume and the nature of the problem. The first two points are closely related. If a client is in a deep crisis or is in severe pain, they are more likely to need guidance, a targeted, grounding treatment and the trust that they will receive help. If they have never learned to take responsibility themselves or have no sense of themselves, it is just as necessary for the practitioner to take the lead and do what the client needs according to their perception and expertise. And there are certainly also very tangible, more physical problems in the Shiatsu context that require expert, targeted action.

And yet there are stumbling blocks and situations in Shiatsu that require a different attitude and different behaviour. If the client sees the practitioner predominantly as an expert who will hopefully solve their problem, they adopt a childlike attitude. They become passive, dependent, and, like a child, eager to please the practitioner, avoid negative evaluations, and do everything right. They hand the responsibility for the process over to the practitioner without contributing themselves. All of this makes real contact very difficult.

What makes the contact even more difficult is the following: The child role, in which one is exposed (at least in one's own perception) to the assessments, evaluations and advice of the practitioner, often touches on old hurts from one's own childhood. The client is on guard, projections occur and the contact is disrupted or never established.

So what can we do? Central for me is something that the Danish family therapist Jasper Juul calls equal dignity. Even if I, as a practitioner, take the lead in certain areas, this does not detract from the equal dignity and value of both participants. If I can convey this attitude authentically, the client may be open to guidance and targeted action without feeling looked down upon.

However, one of the aims of Shiatsu – at least as I see it – is to open up more and more space for self-awareness, self-regulation and personal responsibility as far as the client is able to go. And the more this happens, the more both client and practitioner are in contact with themselves, their dignity and their potential, the sooner a real encounter at eye level is possible.

About Empathy, Centring und Reflective Distance

It just feels good to be seen, to be understood. We have all experienced this. To understand another person, you need a skill that Carl Rogers, the founder of the client-centred psychotherapy approach emphasised: empathy, the ability to cognitively and emotionally put yourself in another person's shoes and to communicate what you have perceived in them.

Can you have too much empathy? As with Yin and Yang, for every pole there is an opposite pole that demands its right. If my attention is so focused on the other person that I merge with them, I can easily lose myself and there is no boundary between me and the other. »Without a boundary, there is no touch«, says Mechthild Erpenbrecht in this context.

Touch occurs at the boundary between me and you, physically through the skin, but also energetically or emotionally. However, we should not imagine this boundary to be too rigid. Again, it is a matter of oscillating between a state in which I am completely with myself and a deep connection with the other person.

In a workshop, Joachim Schrievers, a Shiatsu and Qigong teacher from Bissingen/Teck, Germany, once suggested an exercise that I would like to share with you here in part:

> Two people, one in the role of the practitioner, the other in the role of the client, held each other by the hand. The practitioner focused his attention entirely on himself and his feelings. The client was out of sight. After a while, he changed the focus of attention. He was now completely with the client and did not pay any attention to himself at all. In a third phase, the focus of attention settled in an area that felt right for the situation and for both partners.
> This was a fascinating experience for me. I still remember it vividly. On the outside, nothing was happening, but energetically I could definitely feel where the practitioner's attention was.
> When his attention was elsewhere, I myself felt somehow rigid, left alone and cold.

My colour sensation was grey. When he was completely with me, I felt like a child being watched closely and had no space of my own. I took cover to keep a bit of privacy. My muscles tensed and my breathing accelerated. Only when the right amount of attention was balanced out for both of us was I able to relax and get involved. My experience in the role of the practitioner in this exercise was also revealing. When I focused all my attention on myself and my issues, I also felt rather cool, mechanical, and less in the flow. When I focused all my attention on my partner, it became exhausting for me. And I would involuntarily tense my muscles to avoid »falling into« my partner. There was also a certain fear of being »sucked in« and being drawn into a vortex.

It seems to make sense for us as practitioners to take a reflective distance from what is happening, a bird's eye view so to speak. This allows us to observe from a higher perspective what we are empathically experiencing in ourselves or in the client. We can regulate the direction in which the pendulum should swing between connection and disconnection, we have the opportunity to regulate the emotions triggered by empathy and we get an idea of how to understand the current process. I sometimes imagine this bird's eye view with its perspective from a reflective distance as a stunt kite, a stunt kite that is firmly connected to me and my centre.

When the practitioner is in good contact with their own centre and deep peace, they can compassionately absorb the client's vibrations with all that is difficult, without being thrown off balance. And perhaps then something becomes possible that the psychoanalyst Wilfred Bion calls Containing: from this deeply centred place of peace, the practitioner can absorb what may be unbearable for the client, transform it into something more bearable and peaceful within and then return it to the client through resonance.

When this happens, a connection on a deeper level arises between practitioner and client.

After everything we have looked at so far, it becomes clear how crucial the inner alignment of the practitioner is for an authentic connection to be possible. As important as expert knowledge and techniques are at a certain level, what is fundamental for an encounter is not what you know, but what you are.

What to do? (Hotline to the Inner Observer)

How can I become aware of my own attitudes, actively change them or establish new ones? What supports me in taking a reflective distance from time to time and adopting a bird's eye view? How do I stay in deep contact with myself and my centre? In both Eastern and Western traditions, there are various practices that can help with this, for example Zen and Vipassana meditation, Taiji, Qigong, Yoga from the East, Psychosynthesis and Focusing from the West, and Mindfulness-Based Stress Reduction (MBSR) by Jon Kabat-Zinn, which integrates various traditions. Despite all the differences, what these approaches have in common is the training of mindfulness and the promotion of a connection to an inner observer. The observer is an instance within us that perceives in a completely neutral way how and what we observe, according to which concepts we interpret what we observe, which feelings, inner images and bodily reactions arise. It creates a free space, a distance from the observed content. It prevents us from identifying with certain perceptions, interpretations or reactions and enables us to be equanimous, accepting and flexible in our reactions to changing situations. This observer cannot himself be the object of our observation, he is not a little man in our mind, but first of all an auxiliary construct to give this meta-level position a name and a framework of understanding. The Philosopher Ken Wilber refers to the observer as the »Witness« and warns:

> »So the first mistake is that people sabotage the Witness by trying to make it an object that can be grasped, whereas it is simply the Seer of all objects that arise, and it is ›felt‹ only as a great background sense of Freedom and Release from all objects.«

The Witness, the observer as background noise, as a state of consciousness …

A more physical approach to the inner observer can be found through a phenomenon that Eugene Gendlin, the founder of Focusing, called Felt Sense. The Felt Sense is the physical sensation that arises in connection with a certain situation, a question or a problem. It is not a mental but a physical act, a comprehensive, unclear feeling about a situation, similar to a person's aura. The Felt Sense can also contain important messages for me when I ask questions into it and bring initially unclear aspects into consciousness: How do I feel in this treatment? What image of the situation as a whole emerges in me? Where does the process want to go? What need do I perceive in myself?

Our observer is also called upon in another area: even if we would like to reject it for rational reasons or reasons of professional ethics, in practice it happens again and again that a client or the whole process upsets, irritates or fascinates us, or that we simply don't like the client.

And just like that, the connection is severed. The first step is to be aware of this and admit it, which is an important start. In order to learn to deal with this, we can then direct the spotlight of our awareness to an area that C.G. Jung called the Shadow. The Shadow is the part of our soul that absorbs all the parts of our personality that contradict our positive self-image, that we dislike about ourselves, that are not socially accepted. It is a rich source of stumbling blocks in dealing with ourselves and other people, because what we do not accept in ourselves, we perceive all the more acutely in the outside world and get inflamed by it. It is therefore highly worthwhile to pay attention to our personal shadow from time to time, in the context of coaching, psychotherapy or dream work, for example.

The fundamental thing is not what you know, but what you are. This is how the previous section of this essay concluded. In order for our Shiatsu treatments to become a fruitful encounter, in addition to techniques and expert knowledge we need a lifelong development of ourselves as human beings on various levels, of energetic perception, mindfulness, awareness of the images and concepts that shape our perception and also of our shadow parts. Practices such as meditation, Qigong, Yoga, Psychosynthesis and Focusing can all be helpful.

»What lofty demands«, some people will now sigh and tense their shoulders. No, the suggestions in this essay are by no means intended as contributions to therapist superego, but rather as points of reference that we can approach step by step, each at our own pace, according to our own needs and our own possibilities.

External Practice – Behaviour Reflects Attitude

The inner attitude of the practitioner has a direct effect on the relationship with the client through resonance, regardless of how they present themselves to the outside world. I am quite sure about that, which is why I have devoted so much time to the subject. But how do the attitudes described above manifest themselves outwardly, and what behaviours might run counter to them? In the following, I will pose some questions to raise awareness of the alignments and contradictions between the inner and outer realms.

- The relationship that I am consciously or unconsciously establishing with my client is already evident from our position in the room. Does the practitioner sit behind a desk, separated from the client, during the pre/post talk? Does the session start with both sitting or immediately with the client lying down and the practitioner sitting next to them in a higher position? Is the client asked where in the room the practitioner should be? All this says a lot about eye level, equal dignity and expert status.

- What messages does the room design send? Are there many meridian charts on the wall or are there certificates that document the expert status of the practitioner? Is the room set up to make the client feel welcome? Does it look more like a doctor's office or more like a meditation room? What colours predominate? What does it smell like? Is there a drink available?

- How am I dressed as practitioner? In therapist's white or in everyday clothes?

- After the diagnosis, do I mentally create a treatment plan and follow it consistently, unperturbed by any deviations in the process?

- Do I refer to my notes from previous treatments to provide some continuity to the treatment series, or do I approach each treatment with a fresh perspective?

- Do I communicate my diagnoses and observations in clear language or in creative ambiguity that allows for interpretation?

- Do I invite the client to talk about personal experiences, feelings, and problems, or do I keep the treatment purely on an energetic level?

- Can I allow long periods of silence or inactivity?

- To what extent do I adapt to the client's needs and wishes? To what extent do I keep an eye on my own needs?

- Do I pay sufficient attention to my own energetic and emotional well-being?

From my perspective, there are no clear right or wrong answers to these questions. The respective contexts are too varied. What's more important is to ask yourself these questions from time to time and to be aware of their importance in shaping relationships.

Encounter and Intention?

»Finding Authentic Connection« is the title of this essay. You may have got the impression that encounters are perfectly feasible, that they will happen automatically if only all the factors mentioned are sufficiently taken into account. Not at all! The client may simply say »Leave again!« (at least inwardly), like Lukas from the institution for disabled people whom I mentioned in the beginning. Whether we find and authentic connection or not is not in our hands. We can only carefully prepare the field for it. Resonance is beyond our control. As we have already seen, this is one of its characteristics. Or, as Martin Buber puts it:

> »The Thou meets me through grace – it is not found by seeking.«

Addendum

As with everything in life, the attitudes and behaviour of practitioners are subject to polarity. Different things are needed in different contexts. No one pole is right in itself. To enable you to recognise your own tendencies, your own profile and your own possible biases, I have juxtaposed various attitudes and behaviours in a table.

The Yin and Yang of Practitioner Skills

YIN	YANG
Free-Floating Attention	Precise observation
Sensing	Reflection
Going Along with the Process	Leading
Soft, ambiguous language	Directness
Open, receptive, without concept	Targeted, deductive, diagnostic
Creative not knowing	Expertise
Intuitive treatment	Targeted use of techniques
Acknowledging what is	Actively working on change
I-Thou attitude	I-It attitude
Beginner's mind	Expert mind
Empathy	Centring
Compassion	Reflective distance
Humility, acceptance of one's own shortcomings	Self-optimisation
Ressource orientation	Problem orientation
Wait and see	Action

Literature

Bion, Wilfred (2006): *Aufmerksamkeit und Deutung.* Brandes & Aspel.

Buber, Martin (2010): *Ich und Du.* Gütersloher Verlagshaus.

Erpenbeck, Mechthild (2018): *Wirksam werden im Kontakt.* Carl-Auer.

Harrer, Michael E. / Weiss, Halko (2019): *Wirkfaktoren der Achtsamkeit.* Schattauer.

Rosa, Hartmut (2020): *Unverfügbarkeit.* Residenz-Verlag.

Suzuki, Shunryu (1985): *Zen Mind, Beginner's Mind.* WEATHERHILL.

Wilber, Ken (2001): *Einfach »Das«.* Fischer Taschenbuch.

Yulzari, Rami: *Im Freiraum.* In: Shiatsu-Journal 089/2017.

2

Heidy van Koesveld

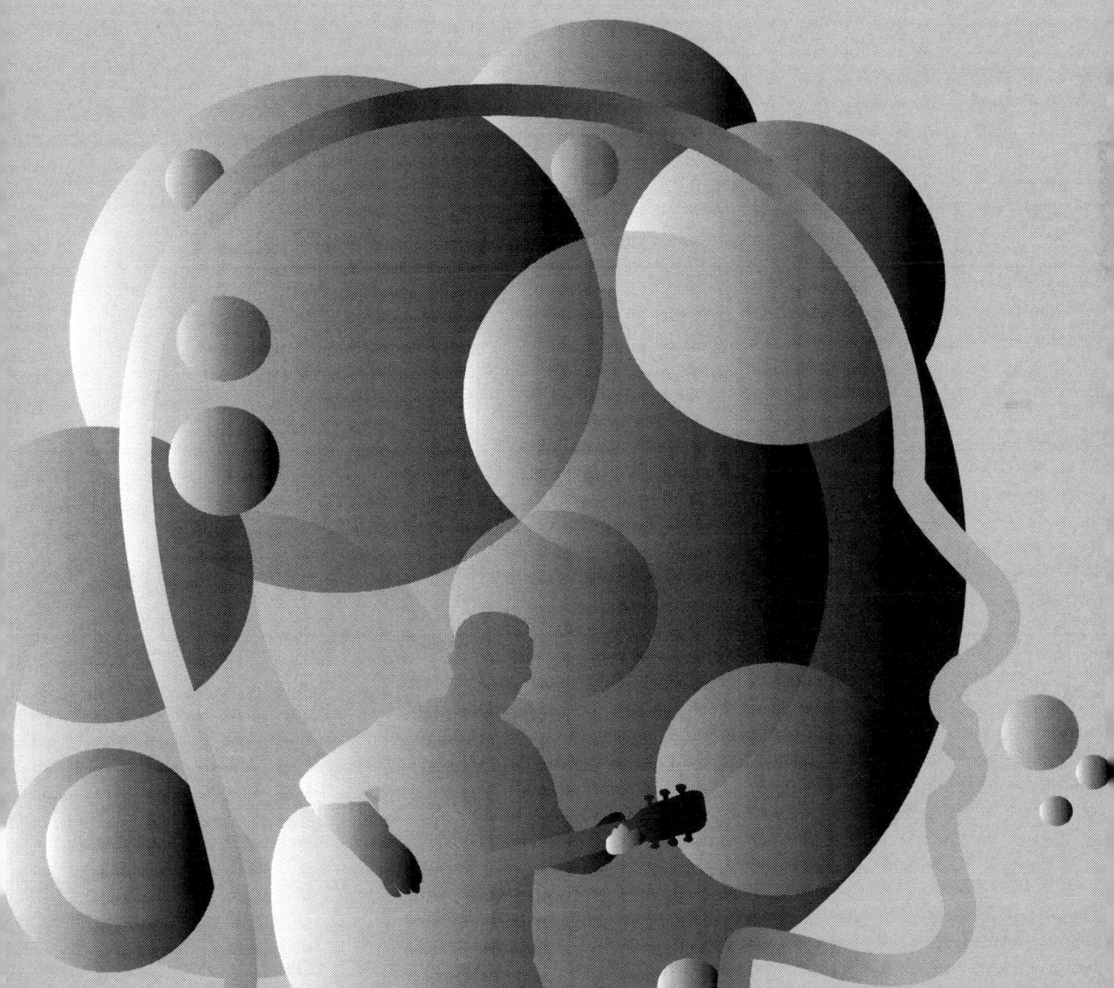

DJ

"Fine tuning, wonderful craft ...

Everybody is born with preferences. We all know more or less by nature what we want.

Sometimes this clarity can be blurred, but when it comes to the simple things in life, we do know. Pasta or rice? Biking or walking? High heels or trainers? What's the food that you can always find in your fridge?

And what about music?! You have a natural taste for rhythm, volume, beats per minute, instrumental or solo, and this is only just about music! The tune that you go well with you recognise immediately. It doesn't really make a difference if these are heavy metal riffs or syllabic Gregorian chanting. You just have to hear a few notes and you recognise it and relax.

For instance (like me), you've been a sucker for Motown music for as long as you can remember. Good old soul with a nice groove … You pick it up through an open window on a busy street and your ear wants to lean into it. You listen to it when you're confused or sad and you put it on like a comfy pair of old jeans. Know what I mean? I think this is all about your personal soundtrack. Your own Motown.

Of course, your personal soundtrack is flexible and will adjust to life's circumstances. Sometimes you want more action, something different, a new tone. Fortunately, your soundtrack covers all of this because of its diversity of tracks. But there might be a time when you don't know what your Motown is at that moment. Too much switching, too much listening to other people's playlist, turning the volume up and down or still listening to your parent's idols. Then you may not even realise that what you're listening to is no longer your own personal tune.

In my practice I sometimes see people come in with the volume turned down to almost zero. Or someone who used to be devoted to Engelbert Humperdinck now only hears techno trance in their head all the time. How would it be if you could hear your Motown but only in slow motion? What has happened? It can have lots of different causes but it doesn't really matter. How lovely would it be to rediscover your own tune of this moment and to be able to unwind within its embrace in it?

As a shiatsu therapist, I tend to feel like a DJ with a beautiful, state-of-the-art mixing console and shelves full of lovely music. What's someone's personal tune? What makes someone happy? When does the body start to move effortlessly? What kind of style, more bass, a little less filtering, just the right volume. You get a soft smile, you cry because you haven't heard that tune for such a long time or you get inspired and start making new plans. Which tune makes you recognise your own soundtrack and feel at home again?

When we've done this heartfelt listening, seeing, hearing and finally found just the right tune, we both feel that there's an endless understanding between us. No need for words, as if we are nodding our heads in sync to the newly found tune.

This kind of fine-tuning makes me endlessly inquisitive and gives my own Motown the exact the right pace.

Fine tuning, wonderful craft …

3

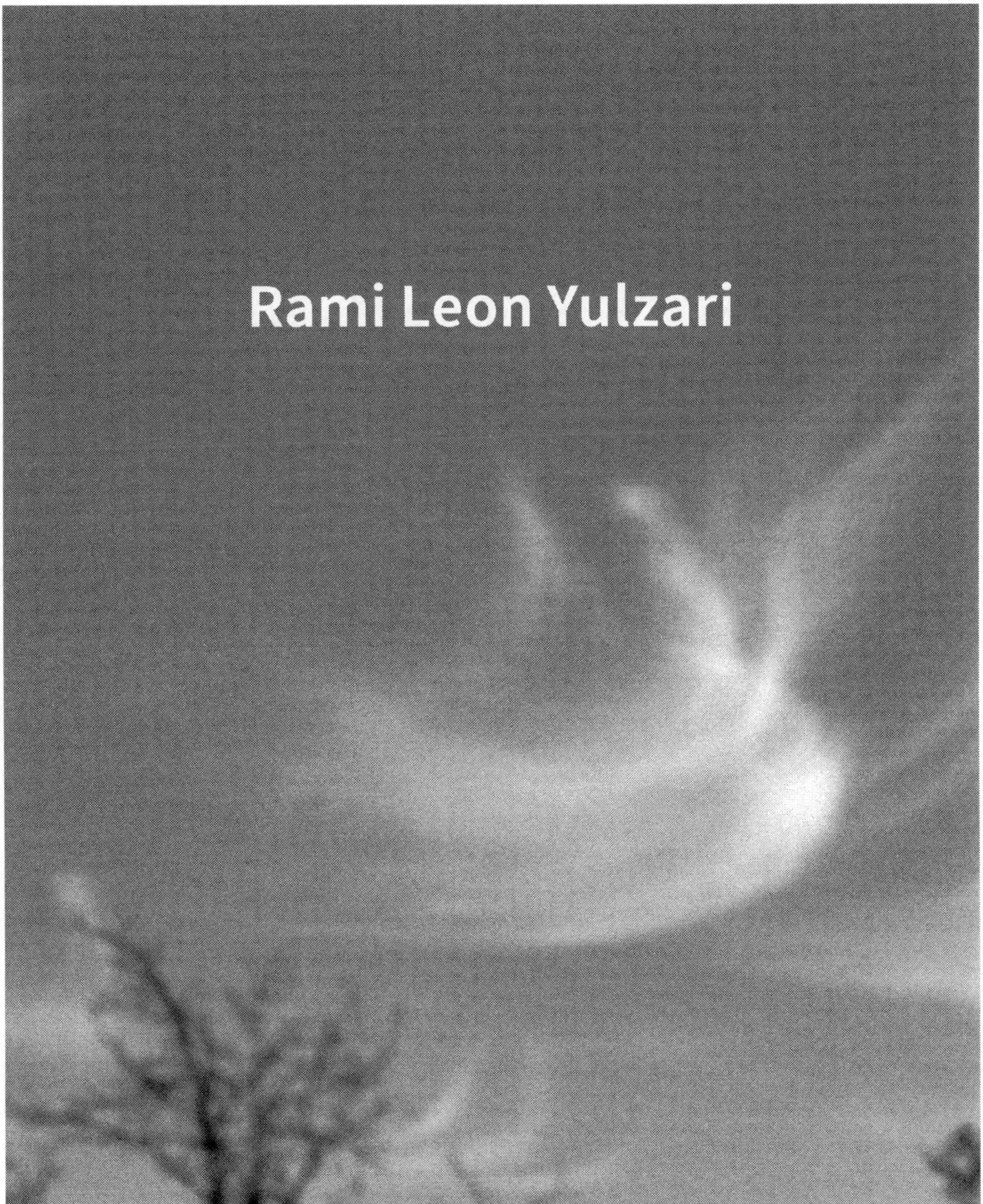

Being in Suspension

”Suspending allows us to see what we have not seen before, or have not seen clearly. We find in the patient and in ourselves the possibility to stay and to endure. What was once urgent and unbearable is now suspended, a safe space in which to linger.

»Hurry, please. Put a bandage on my heart when you put me to bed« is a line from Ehud Banai's[1] song »Hurry, please«. The song tells the story of a thirty-year-old son, sick with fever, without work or love, who returns to sleep on his parents' couch. I have heard the song many times, but recently, as sometimes happens when the wing of a stray pigeon hits the windscreen, I began to pay attention to the lyrics. A thirty-year-old son turns to his mother and says, »Please hurry. I am hurt. My heart is wounded«. He begs her to apply a bandage to stop the bleeding of his wounded heart, to save him from death.

»Hurry, please« is the plea and demand of a person suffering from heartache to his mother to nurse and care for him. He wants to be relieved of his suffering. He expects his mother to apply a bandage. Will applying a bandage stop the bleeding? Will it heal the wound? Of course not. Nevertheless, applying a bandage is a deliberate and healing act.

I remember another bandage

I was a young soldier in the Sinai desert during the Yom Kippur War[2]. The sun was shining that day; the sand was blindingly yellow. Volley after volley of artillery rained down from the clear blue sky. Then it was quiet. The desert was silent. People emerged from all sides and looked around. It seemed that no one had been hurt until we saw the damage to the ambulance at the side of the road. There was a driver and a paramedic inside. They looked fine through the windscreen, but as I approached I saw that the driver was wounded, his torn abdomen exposing bleeding internal organs.

I find myself sitting next to his stretcher, which had been placed on a half-track for evacuation. The paramedic at his feet tries in vain to find a blood vessel into which to inject morphine. He calls the injured man's name, reminds him of the baby born to him the week before, and begs him to stay with us. A religious soldier holding the stretcher handles recites »Shema Israel«[3] loudly, over and over – his way of announcing the presence of death. The wounded man mumbles »water« and the medic tells me to just wet his lips. I try. The paramedic tells me to apply a bandage. I still remember tearing the plastic wrapping off the bandage, my hands

1 Ehud Banai is an Israelian singer and songwriter.

2 1973 war

3 »The Lord is our God, the Lord is one.« Jews traditionally recite the Shema prayer as their last words.

shaking as I tried to apply the bandage to the intestines, gently so as not to cause pain – a white sailboat floating in an ocean of blood.

Since then I have known that applying a bandage is a symbolic act, a ritual, a kind of prayer, like straightening a child's blanket before they go to sleep.

As a Shiatsu therapist, instead of a bandage, I lay my hand, a hand that wants to be big and warm and bring comfort. Laying a hand is a symbolic act and at the same time it is the thing itself; one hand is laid on the patient, the other follows. These hands carry the possibility of change, the possibility of healing, the possibility of carrying the burden when it has become unbearable. Hands touch pain. Sometimes they are more like a bandage applied to a void.

Hurry, please, the pain is great, the fear of pain is unbearable. The fear that clings to pain is deceptive – if the pain goes away, the suffering will go away. The longing for its disappearance creates the dream of immediate release. Concentrating on his fears, on the pain that grows and accumulates until his whole being is defined by this core pain, the patient wants to be released immediately. This is the salvation of the good mother, the breastfeeding mother, the mother who instantly responds to her baby's needs; a nipple to the mouth puts an end to hunger and fear, leads back to beneficial, comforting warmth.

The dream of instant redemption in our culture is fed by drugs, painkillers, antidepressants and psychedelics – medicine on the one hand and mystical experience on the other. In our dream, pain disappears instantly. In our dream, everyone can eliminate suffering at any time.

With the memory of the nursing mother and the image of the healer, magician or sorcerer, the patient comes to the clinic with the message: I'm scared, quickly, relieve my pain.

Knowing that he has no magic wand, that he cannot conjure up medical magic, what can the therapist do?

He suspends. He holds the hand of the restless, anxious patient and offers him the chance to slow down. Slowness takes the physical, mental and emotional movement out of our daily behaviour, out of our habits. Then we can examine, delving slowly and gradually into the details. We stop and rest on a bench by the road and have a look at the landscape before moving on.

In his book »Rediscovering Psychoanalysis«, Thomas Ogden describes a meeting he attended where a group of doctors were discussing the psychological aspects of their work. One doctor recounted an occasion when a patient had left him a message that her mother had died in bed at home. On arriving at the mother's home, he confirmed the death and immediately called an ambulance. »Why did you do that?« the moderator asked. Startled by the question, the doctor replied: »Because she was dead«. The moderator then asked: »Why not sit down with the daughter for a cup of tea?«

For Ogden, sitting down for a cup of tea means keeping options open: »Allowing for what must happen to happen. Sitting down for a cup of tea means allowing the event to stay beyond time for a moment.«

I remember when my own mother died; it took a while before they came for her body. It was early one ordinary day and my mother was in bed, but that morning she did not get up. Death had already taken her. Time was both full and empty. There was a silence between people, protected by the silence of my dead mother. I remember the blossoming branch of an almond tree. A moment of grace.

Ogden writes: »The question why not sit down for a cup of tea, made me feel the need for designing a space in which there is time, dream-time, where people can experience something together and dream it together. What can happen in this space is unique to the situation and people living it.«

»Please hurry. Put a bandage on my heart when you put me to bed.« Once I'm asleep you won't be able to take care of me – I'll be in another world, the world of sleep and dreams, a world to which you have no access. This world is private, hidden even from the healing mother, the saviour. If the injury enters the world of sleep and dreams, it will become a part of it. It may be too late. Is there no healing for the wounded heart in the dream world?

In quiet suspension, ›dream time‹, the therapist may find his or her mind wandering. The source of the wandering can be either the patient, lost in thoughts and feelings and perhaps even dozing off, or the therapist, present and at the same time wandering in his or her thoughts, floating in their feelings.

Thomas Ogden describes this state as daydreaming or reverie (from the French word rêve, meaning dream). »This was not a mere coincidence that his thoughts wandered«, he writes in his book »On Not Being Able to Dream«. The therapist talks to himself inwardly, privately. It is a natural act, carried out automatically and unconsciously, which deals with the most personal of things.

Modes of reverie, says Ogden, are not a reflection of inattention. On the contrary, they express a sense of the patient's experience that cannot yet be formulated or even felt. According to Ogden, what appears to be an escape from the effort of being present and attentive to the patient instead becomes a significant and perhaps essential part of the patient's experience.

A Zen Shiatsu therapist walks the path of Zen, the path of meditation, the path of self-emptying. Attention is focused on the patient, who becomes the object of meditation. The Zen-Shiatsu therapist may occasionally find himself relaxing his posture and concentration. If his thoughts wander, he has an anchor – his body anchor – which touches the patient's body. From there he can take off, move away and come back again.

My first experience of such a reverie is etched in my memory: I put my hand on a patient's stomach and found myself deep in the sea, floating in dark water among fish and vegetation. What had begun as a possibility of peace and tranquillity became instead frightening and disturbing. I had touched horror.

To the state of reverie, of the mind wandering aimlessly, the therapist adds intention. Intention allows us to catch the tails of wandering thoughts and anchor them in a therapeutic context. Whether they come from the therapist or the patient, these thoughts and feelings are creations of the therapeutic context, where two people meet and influence each other.

The Shiatsu therapist, attentive to his patient's qi, adds intentionality to his attentiveness. At the same time, he is attuned to his own qi and to the connection thus created between himself and the patient. The qigong practitioner is attentive to the movement of qi within and to the expression of movement when it meets qi from the outside. Shiatsu treatment and Qi-Gong practice are both involved in the same process; listening to Qi with intention.

The term used to describe our awareness while practicing qigong is called Yi-Nien. The first part of this term is Yi, which means intention or awareness. The second part, Nien, is what comes from thinking. I call Yi-Nien Gentle Attention.

In full attention we focus our awareness on a particular object, whether it is a physical process such as breathing or a mental object, thought or image. It could even be something that exists between the physical and mental levels, such as pain in a particular place. When we focus our full attention, our awareness focuses on an object, studying it, seeing it in increasing detail with greater emotional or sensory quality. Focusing our awareness in this way allows us to move outside our usual barrage of thoughts, the everyday noise. We silence the ›monkey mind‹.

Gentle Attention, on the other hand, is focused on several objects at once, moving freely and smoothly from one object to another without pause. Practice and experience allow us to experience Gentle Attention as an uninterrupted sequence, to suspend without getting stuck.

In full attention we see more and more detail as our vision becomes more precise and focused. In Gentle Attention our seeing sees and does not see. It is a floating vision.

Professor Jiao writes in his book »Health Care through Qi-Gong«: »The directive is that Yi-Nien should be as it is – as it is not«. In this situation the usual separation between what is physical, emotional, sensory or conscious disappears. We move and Yi-Nien accompanies our movement – as if someone who is us also accompanies us. Yi-Nien becomes double vision; we see and are seen at the same time. In this state we are transformed. Like the roses in T.S. Eliot's »Four Quartets«: »... for the roses had the look of flowers being looked at.«[4]

In Gentle Attention the therapist can make »lack of attention« the object of his attention. He constantly examines how fluctuations in his own qi – his body and mind, feelings and emotions – relate to the movements of his patient's qi. Gentle Attention then serves as both a diagnostic and therapeutic tool, since treatment and diagnosis are always simultaneous.

When the therapist recognizes sensations in his sensory organ – his qi – he will be able to harness those that relate to the patient's diagnosis. When this happens, it becomes possible to ›go with the feeling‹ and find out where the spontaneous movement created by the patient's qi might lead. Therapeutic movement derived from Gentle Attention will be gentle, attentive, supportive, sequential and targeted.

As the patient's qi becomes the source of sensation, movement is created in the therapist's qi, which can then be returned to the patient. The therapist will accompany and support the movement of qi, with the basic assumption that the essential purpose of qi movement is always to seek balance.

---

[4] Eliot, T.S. (2015): *Vier Quartette.* Bibliothek Suhrkamp, S. 11.

Suspension creates a pause, a space between things, what the Japanese call *Mah*. *Mah* is the space between each and every thing on a macro or micro level. We might imagine that space to be empty; that it contains nothing and is completely still. But if we stay in between, we find that space is full and in constant motion. Unlike a fractal image – where even though we witness constant change, we find infinite identical structures contained in every detail – qi is life. Life is movement, and you cannot step into the same river twice.

And what is there in *Mah*? Qi. The sense of qi is the most primitive level, the primary level of our feelings, our first communication with ourselves and the world around us. Qi is energy in the sense of vitality. It includes our thoughts and consciousness, as well as our physical and emotional sensations. In this sense the word energy refers to the pre-verbal sensory world where there is no separation, where all is one.

The initial feeling is loaded with meaning; a feeling that comes from an undifferentiated source – a movement in an organ, a thought, an emotion, a sight, sound or smell. Once absorbed, we can try to identify the source and analyze it in terms of detection, decoding, propagation, shape, form or connection theory. However, the primary essence of qi is neither the body nor the mind, but an undifferentiated sense organ within the human being.

We can feel qi both in close physical contact and from a distance. We can feel our own qi, the qi of another person, or even the qi of a room, whether that room is empty or filled with objects or people.

With practice, we can train this sensory organ and increase its receptive capacity. The receptive mode becomes a state of wakefulness that comes from the stillness of deep meditation. Waking is not necessarily vigilance; it can take the form of daydreaming or reverie, a kind of floating somnolence in which the qi is not focused on a particular organ or place.

Full attention is an act of awareness and works best when the body is put aside, when feelings of pain, hunger and thirst are eliminated. Gentle attention senses a fundamental vibration, a primal sound, or, in Ogden's words, registers a sense of experience that cannot yet be formulated or even felt. Remaining in this state and receiving a sensation, the therapist responds.

At its best, this communication is two-way and reciprocal. Just as another's breath affects our own, so our breath affects another's. Mutuality is created, beginning with influence and continuing to gradually dissolve all separation. It should be noted, of course, that entering into this mode is somewhat different for the patient and the therapist. The therapist guides the therapeutic process. He can recognise the signs of qi imbalance in the reverie and thereby support the patient's movement towards balancing the qi.

Attentive to Qi, the therapist seeks *Mah*; that which is in-between and unknown.

And how do we stay in this terrifying unknown?

We suspend

The therapist who suspends, allowing space in between, can continue to apply the bandage even as the patient enters their private world of sleep and dreams.

Suspending allows us to see what we have not seen before, or have not seen clearly. We find in the patient and in ourselves the possibility to stay and to endure. What was once urgent and unbearable is now suspended, a safe space in which to linger?

4

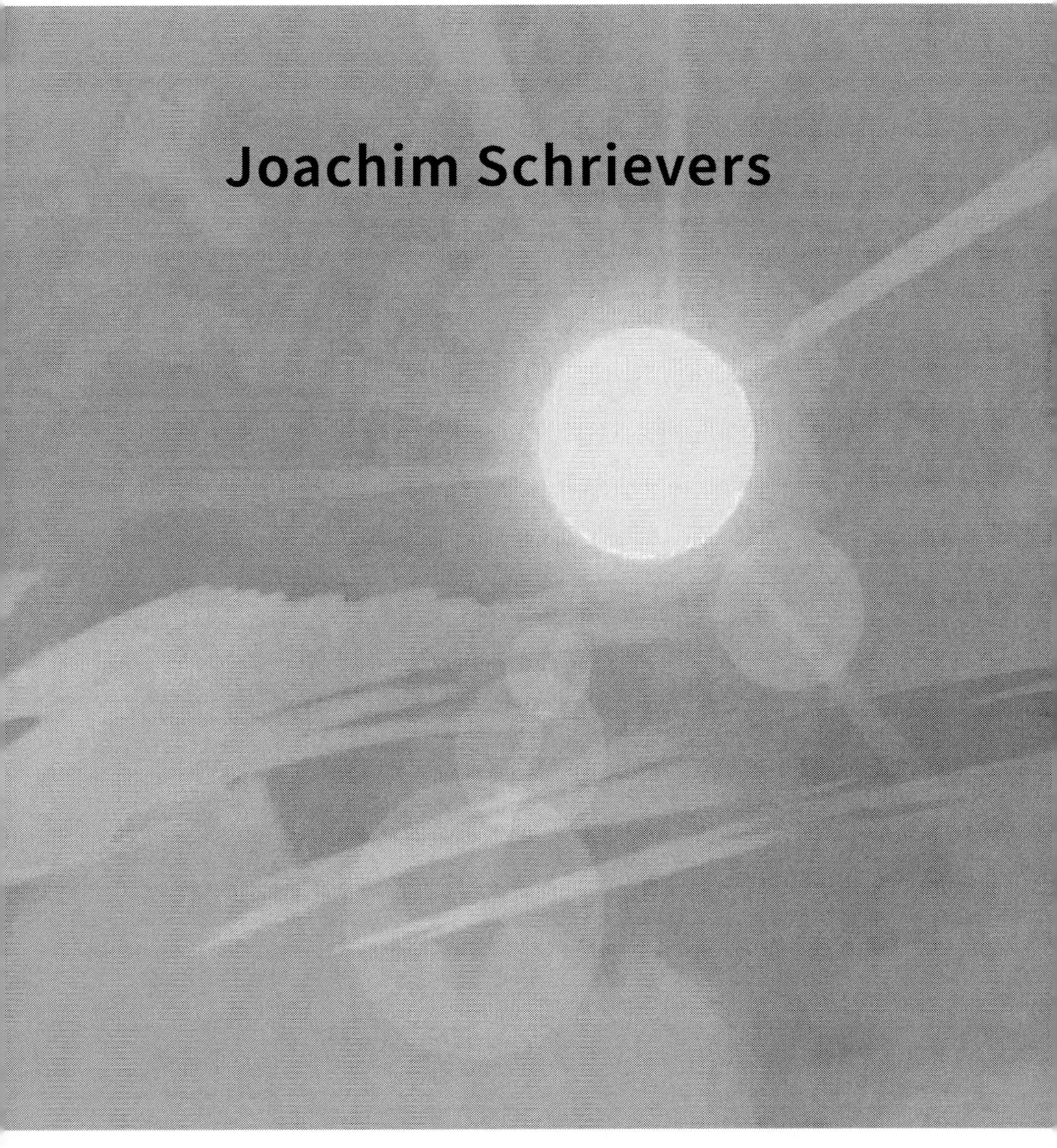

Joachim Schrievers

From Practitioner to Companion

” **While a practitioner is more like a taxi driver, who takes a passenger to a certain destination (e.g., pain relief) without the passenger having to do anything – apart from paying – a companion works as a driving instructor, with the aim of not only showing the way but also teaching the passenger how to drive the car. The most important tool in this process is the training of attention, through which the client learns to relate to their own inner experiences.**

A few years, ago, a friend of mine called me and told me that she had a slipped disc in her lumbar spine, and that her doctor had recommended surgery, for which she had already made an appointment at a clinic. She asked me if I knew of any treatment options that could help her avoid an operation. I recommended a nearby acupuncture centre that works with the support of competent and experienced visiting Chinese doctors. It wasn't long before she called me again to inform me that a miracle had happened. Her symptoms had disappeared after the first treatment. On the advice of her doctors, she received nine further treatments to stabilise her condition and had cancelled the operation.

However, several things had disturbed her: Firstly, each time she was seen by a different doctor, who, after the usual pulse and tongue diagnosis, inserted the needles and then left her alone until the needles were removed. No one wanted to know anything about her beyond her symptoms, and she didn't feel involved in the treatment process. As a young woman with two small children, she had lost her husband to suicide, something she was always painfully aware of, including during the time before the disc herniation. At the acupuncture centre, she felt very competently treated but not accompanied.

Although this example is not specifically related to Shiatsu, a similar scenario could occur in the context of Shiatsu. The client describes their symptoms or general state of health, and the Shiatsu practitioner, using their knowledge and experience, selects points, meridians, and techniques to improve the client's condition. The client, as in the case of my friend, simply has the task of lying down and allowing the treatment to unfold. If we understand Shiatsu as a form of companionship, however, the role of the client changes: they are no longer passive but become active participants. They not only take part in in their own process but gradually learn to control and influence it.

Shiatsu also opens up other possibilities. The intense time spent together in silence and contemplation can lead to moments of deep self-awareness. Self-awareness here means that the client sometimes experiences themselves in a completely new way during the *therapeutic state*: in lightness or leaden heaviness, filled with creative urge or in bottomless fatigue, brimming over with well-being or touched by unpleasant memories. These experiences, ranging from the perception of the physical realm to transpersonal experiences of one's own boundlessness in time and space, can be greatly enriching. We know that our energy system contains a wide variety of forces – some of which are common to all of us, part of being human, while others are related to our personal experiences. Memories of beautiful events in our lives can become an inexhaustible source of strength, but life force can also be bound up in unresolved traumatic experiences and thus no longer freely available to us, restricting our development.

Such self-awareness often emerges spontaneously, more often in some people and less often or not at all in others. It brings into the client's consciousness something that was previously hidden in the unconscious. In the silence and receptivity of a Shiatsu treatment, we encounter feelings that need to be felt, experiences that need to be lived and forces that need to be integrated. In Shiatsu, we cannot encounter anything that does not belong to us in some way. It is precisely, when we do not consciously seek or try to provoke specific experiences with certain techniques, when they arise naturally, that it becomes clear that there is a kind of innate drive towards wholeness, healing and integration in all of us. When a Shiatsu treatment leads to an intense self-contact, the client, or more precisely, the conscious self, is automatically involved in the process – and since many people have no previous experience of this, they then need guidance.

In addition to these processes, there are also clients who primarily seek guidance or companionship. This means that the client wants to find their own way and is looking for support from another person. They are not looking for someone to do something for them, but for someone to help them do something for themselves. They want to develop competence in dealing with themselves and with life. The question is, to what extent Shiatsu can contribute to such an acquisition of self-competence.

Some may initially think of accompanying exercises that the practitioner gives to the client as homework. I will come to this later. I would like to begin with the experience of Shiatsu itself. Common experiences during and after Shiatsu treatments are, for example, feelings of relaxation, comfortable heaviness or lightness. However, when we look closely, the experience is different for each person. This depends on many different factors, including the current mood, temperament and idiosyncrasies of the client, and last but not least, their entire biography that has shaped them and their self-perception. People come to Shiatsu because it makes them feel good or because it has a positive effect on their complaints and ailments. They are pleased with the results but do not ask themselves what the effective treatment factors might be. They are familiar with the usual explanations, such as improved flow of energy in the meridians and released blockages, and equipped with this knowledge, they surrender to the hands of the practitioner and take a break from everyday life. A particularly deep experience of Shiatsu is often described as being »completely gone«.

We have all experienced that we do not necessarily perceive identical situations and activities in the same way. A day at the seaside, a walk through blossoming orchards or a climb up a mountain are never quite the same, even if it's the same sea, the same orchard and the same mountain. When we are dealing with the loss of a close family member, for example, or are faced with a seemingly insurmountable task at work, we have less room to enjoy our surroundings. People who have fallen into a state of depression or burnout invariably describe how they can no longer vividly experience situations that they used to enjoy, that energised them. They feel empty and apathetic. They have lost the vibrant presence that is a prerequisite for an enjoyable and nourishing experience. Instead, they ruminate on all sorts of things and their thoughts go round in circles. If they can find their way back from thinking and brooding to the path of sensory experience, enjoyment returns, and the ability to draw strength from everyday experience is restored.

But what applies to a pleasant hike also applies to a Shiatsu treatment. Part of the experience comes from external conditions, the landscape, the weather, the treatment. The other part of the experience depends on the internal conditions of the client. Guidance in Shiatsu aims to improve these internal conditions and to show ways in which the client can actively participate. This includes access to internal resources and sources of strength as well as improved grounding and centring.

If we give the same treatment to ten clients in a row – as consistently as possible – and then ask them about their subjective experience, we will receive ten different descriptions. This is not because we provided different treatments after the diagnostic findings, but because the respective internal conditions of the clients were different. Even if we perform the same treatment on one of our clients ten times and ask them about their experience each time, we will observe that they or their Ki reacts differently to the treatments. The differences can be very subtle or quite obvious, since the internal conditions of this one client are different each time.

During a treatment, the client is interested in the practitioner's diagnosis and assessment to understand what is wrong with them. If we understand Shiatsu more as companionship, the roles change: the practitioner is more interested in the client's inner experience in order to better understand them and accompany them in their process. In addition to feeling energetic processes with their hands, dialogue plays a more important role. As an experienced practitioner, we may perceive energetic blockages, but what we don't yet know is how the client feels in their body or what their sense of self is. When we ask the client at the end of a Shiatsu treatment how they feel in their body, in their legs, in their pelvis, and what sensations they are experiencing, it not only gives us information about them but also has another very significant effect: Our question invites them to turn their attention to their internal bodily processes. Trying to find words for their experience leads to an increased awareness of their own sensations, which makes it easier for them to remember the experience, in a similar way to a dream that we remember more easily when we tell someone about it or write it down. Asking about the inner experience prevents the client from »disappearing« completely. As pleasurable as the feeling of being »completely gone« may be, it is only of limited help in coping with our daily lives. Coping with our lives requires our presence, our awareness. This doesn't just mean mental alertness and concentration but physical presence and mindfulness that combines awareness of self, others, and situations. Both the practitioner and the client are primarily interested in the experience – the changes that occur such as pain reduction are welcomed as »side effects«.

Sensitivity develops from the process of perception. Our attitude to life, whether we are happy or unhappy, is something that is made up of subtle and the refined body signals; it is something that we sense or feel. Our modern, technologically advanced society with its mental overload and physical degeneration, brings with it a disconnection from our inner experience, which is also a physical experience. This has serious consequences because our body awareness is a crucial aspect of the self-regulation of our organism and our psyche.

Take hunger, for example. Hunger is a bodily sensation that prompts us to correct an imbalance, such as low blood sugar. By craving something specific, our body not only signals that it needs nourishment but also indicates which nutrients it is lacking. Animals are known to have the ability to eat the herbs whose properties are beneficial to them when they are ill. We humans have largely lost this instinct. This is reflected, for example, in the ever-increasing number of eating disorders. In people with anorexia nervosa, the sense of their own body is so diminished that they feel unattractively fat, even though they are far too thin. It is often a shock for them to see their own body in a photograph, and they can hardly believe that they are that person.

People with Attention Deficit Hyperactivity Disorder (ADHD) often have a very high sensitivity to external stimuli, but a very low awareness of what is going on in their own bodies. They have developed a strong sensitivity to others, but have lost it towards themselves. Their inner experience of physicality, grounding and centring does not provide an adequate counterbalance to the incoming external stimuli. This disorder is also increasing at an alarming rate.

It has already been mentioned that the experience of joy is greatly reduced or lost in burnt-out and depressed people. Joy, like all our emotions and moods, is a bodily experience, as these feelings arise from body signals that are received and interpreted in the brain. It could be said that a loss of self-awareness is a symptom of these illnesses, but it could just as well be that the disorders are the result of alienation from one's own body and the forces at work within it. Ultimately, whether the chicken or the egg came first is secondary; what matters is that people learn to experience themselves alive in their bodies again, to receive the signals the body sends, and to respond to them.

The vivid experience of our body on all levels is the basis for natural self-regulation and self-healing. That which applies to hunger applies equally to all other needs. The need for rest, for social contact, the desire for a concert or a good book are all shaped by signals from the body, that help us do what is good for us and restore our balance. Conversely, our lives can easily become unbalanced if we are unaware of, or consciously ignore, our body's corrective needs and moods. Physical and psychological disorders of various kinds are often the result. When we guide people in Shiatsu to feel their bodies better and more deeply, to be *fully present* instead of absent, we are not treating disorders and illnesses, but strengthening self-regulation and self-healing. We are not the ones doing the work; it is the client's energy system or ki, striving for balance, that does the work.

An image can illustrate the idea of companionship: If we, as listeners, are to be touched and deeply moved at a concert, three components are crucial: the composer, the performer and we the listeners. Without our ability to listen, to be touched and moved, even the greatest musician and the finest music cannot reach us.

In Shiatsu, it's not primarily about our migraine, our liver meridian, or lung ki; it is primarily about us, about how we experience ourselves and how we deal with ourselves and life. When we become »all ears« and learn to feel with our whole body, with our whole energy field, we come into direct contact with life itself.

Thus, it is about introducing our clients to the art of »listening with the whole body«, using all the tools at our disposal in Shiatsu. This listening deepens the impact of our treatment and leads the client to an improved self-awareness, self-efficacy, and self-competence, as well as the ability to follow their own inner flow.

How does this work in practice? After a brief preliminary interview, during which our client describes how they feel and perhaps expresses expectations or wishes, we may ask them to lie down and take some time to arrive. This might be done, for example, in the following manner:

»If you like, you can close your eyes and take some time to fully arrive. Check that you're lying comfortably and that you are vertical! Let your shoulders rest and sink down. Feel the weight of your arms and rest them completely on the mat. Feel your torso from your shoulders to your pelvis. Feel your legs to rest completely on the mat. Now take some time to feel inside and observe how you're doing, how you are feeling. At the end of the treatment, you will have another opportunity to feel inside yourself and compare your experience with the current one. You can use the treatment to feel yourself in every touch, every point and every moment.«

This attunement takes about five minutes, or slightly longer, and helps us to move from the thinking mode to the sensing mode. There are several important aspects to this process. Firstly, it helps the client to relax and calm down as much as possible in the short time available. Calmness is primarily achieved by redirecting attention from the wild activities of the mind (as the ancient Chinese used to say, »the mind is like a horde of wild monkeys«) and focusing on the physical experience. Every practitioner of Qigong experiences something essential after a period of time: Our attention and our Ki follow each other, i.e. when we focus our attention in our shoulders and arms, for example, the energy in that area also increases – more or less depending on our talent and level of practice. This means that the client's body field in that area is strengthened and all natural life movements and functions are gently stimulated and supported. However, this is not the only change initiated by this process. As our body field is also a field of perception, self-perception is trained and improved at the same time, leading to a growing ability to influence internal bodily processes. This is one aspect of self-efficacy. Self-efficacy means that what we do – or refrain from doing – has a noticeable effect. Self-efficacy is a crucial factor in coping with stress because feeling helpless and out of control is stressful for most people.

Let's take the example of a migraine. If we feel tension building up in our shoulders and neck and we know from experience that this is the beginning of a severe migraine attack and that we have no control over it (except perhaps by taking strong medication), we become victims of a dynamic within ourselves, whose origin we do not know. However, if, over time, we experience that our shoulders actually relax and sink as a result of the attunement that precedes the Shiatsu treatment, we begin to realise that we don't have to be mere victims of our inner dynamics, but that there are also natural ways of influencing them, other than chemical ones. Over time, self-efficacy develops into self-competence and a natural ease, and – if we take a conscious interest in these processes – also a new self-image.

The following sentence is deliberately placed at the beginning of the short attunement: »If you like, you may close your eyes and take some time to fully arrive.« It conveys the sense of »I may« (rather than »I must«) and »I have time – as much time as I want or *it* requires«. This is a way of helping our client to get into a receptive state for the treatment. This state is very different from normal waking consciousness. Unlike everyday consciousness, where our attention is almost always directed outwards and we are under time pressure, in the treatment state, our focus turns inwards, and *doing* takes a back seat to *letting* be. The treatment state takes us – depending on its depth – from tension, through relaxation into deep relaxation. The experience of time and its constraining pressure recede, and the sense of confinement and spatial limitation gives way to a sense of vastness and boundlessness. The self begins to surrender to a deeper – or higher – reality. This process is similar to falling asleep. However, unlike falling asleep, where the self surrenders completely to the unconscious and loses consciousness apart for a few remembered dreams, during Shiatsu, the client remains awake. A Shiatsu treatment, in a sense, builds a bridge between the conscious and the unconscious, allowing the client to learn to draw from the richness of the unconscious and discover inner sources of strength. For this to happen, they need to »downshift« but not »switch off«.

The next sentence is:

»Check that you are lying well and align yourself along your vertical axis. Allow your shoulders to relax and sink downwards. Feel the weight of your arms, and rest them completely on the mat.« This invites us to turn our attention to our own body and its inner alignment, to check that it is balanced, both literally and figuratively. It offers a fresh opportunity to »straighten up«.

The client realises that in a moment of reflection, they can better perceive themselves and, if necessary, make small corrections. Behind this seemingly mundane experience lies the fundamental principle of companionship and guidance: that improved self-awareness and self-experience open the possibility for change in alignment with the inherent order of our lives.

At this point I would like to say a few words about the different types of companionship. I live at the foot of a mountain on which there is an old castle, a popular destination for excursions. You can actually see the castle from our house, but many a seminar participant has got lost on the way there. When I accompany the »castle hikers«, that is, walk with them, they naturally reach the top by the shortest route. It is a very natural and straightforward form of companionship. However, it turns out that the attention of the people I accompany varies greatly during the walk. Some, after such a hike, know the path and could find it on their own the next day, while others, concentrating on the beauty of nature or our conversation, have paid so little attention to the path that they would get lost all over again the next day. If I want the people I'm guiding to find their own way in the future, it is a good idea to stop briefly at a fork in the path and consciously draw their attention to it. If they want to know not only the way to the castle but are also to explore other, different paths, then I need to show them how to read a map and use a compass.

The brief preparatory attunement at the beginning of the Shiatsu treatment, means that I can make my client aware of my approach at different stages. If I wish, I can choose to draw attention to the principle behind their experience: the principle of natural correction that comes from pausing and self-awareness or self-experience. Raising this awareness is sometimes, but not always, a good idea – a person entering a good state during the treatment could be torn out of the state of sensing and thrown back into that of thinking. However, this does not necessarily have to be the case. It is a characteristic of a deep treatment state (it would be worth writing an entire book on the quality and importance of the treatment state) that it does not exist *beyond something*, for example, beyond talking and thinking but *in the midst of everything*. It does not belong to the world of »either-or« but to that of »both-and«. It takes us into a world of *inner silence* that does not necessarily require outer silence.

Once a client has learned to enter this inner space, or perhaps inner space-time, this awareness can easily occur during a treatment. On the one hand, it is then closely connected to the experience, and on the other hand, information and insights that reach us in these deep states of treatment can become more deeply embedded in our memory, and thus have a much more lasting effect. For us, as practitioners, there are no patent remedies, but rather changing situations to which we must learn to respond with empathy and sensitivity.

But back to our guided attunement. If we have chosen awareness, we can add the following sentence: »I would like to draw your attention to the step you have just taken. You paused, noticed the position of your body and changed it so that you were more in balance afterwards. You can do that at any time in your daily life.« Our problem is not so much that we don't know what we could or should do – or avoid – for our well-being; our problem is that in the hustle and bustle of our lives we simply forget, or that the path to peace and inwardness seems so far away that we consider it pointless to even try. Entering the treatment state shortens this path. Mind, Ki and body move closer together, what we think becomes an experience, and what we physically experience, we begin to understand.

So, there is a difference between saying this sentence during the attunement phase, when our client is lying with their eyes closed and their attention focused inwards and during the follow-up conversation, when both practitioner and client are back in normal waking consciousness. Applied to our walk to the castle, it would be like discussing the forks and turn-offs with each other after we've reached the top. There would be a significant risk that many important details that are important for remembering the path would already have faded from memory. The guided attunement is like the seed from which the client's own practice is to grow later, and it falls on fertile ground during the treatment state.

But let's continue with the text: »You can let your shoulders rest and allow them to sink. Feel the weight of your arms and let them rest completely on the mat.« Self-awareness or self-contact refers to different aspects and levels of our existence, to the body as well as to energy dynamics within our body. Of course, many people come for Shiatsu who are very sensitive to the energetic processes in their bodies, but the consequences are not always pleasant. People with an open, highly resonant energy field are often more exposed to what is going on around them than those for whom everything seems to bounce off. When they see something unpleasant or feel invisible tensions in the room, »it turns their stomach«, just to give one example of many possible physical reactions. Energetic sensitivity – a real jewel – carries with it the risk of instability, and this is due in part to a lack of grounding. Lack of grounding means that the mind is not really anchored in the body. Our body is the only part of us that has weight and mass; our Ki and our soul weigh nothing. When we invite our clients to feel the weight of their bodies, we help their mind settle into the body. Of course, we always have the same weight on the scale, more or less, but we can only experience it when the field of our attention permeates our body. This is by no means as obvious as one might think. Anyone who has experienced a state of dissociation (»separation«, as opposed to association which implies connection) from the body, knows that it is then barely possible to perceive the simplest of bodily signals, such as the experience of weight. Paradoxically, although, in the end, it is all about the perception of life forces themselves – the experience of lightness, at the beginning it is more about the connection to the body and the experience of heaviness. Just like someone building a tall building, we do well to lay a solid foundation in the ground first.

»Feel your torso from the shoulder girdle to the pelvis and entrust it, together with your legs, completely to the mat.«

As we feel the weight of our body, we also feel the earth beneath us. The invitation to entrust our body to the mat adds a new aspect: trust. When we feel the earth beneath us, literally when we have ground beneath our feet while standing, we connect with something reliable, something that supports us. If we engage with it with our full attention, it can resonate within us, striking the chord of trust that is unconditional, the chord of basic trust. Unlike other mammals, we are born in complete helplessness. But we are also born with the ability to entrust ourselves completely to our mother, father or caregiver. We are born in trust and remain in trust until we experience something that breaks this trust. Our basic needs as newborns are simple: food, warmth and closeness (love and affection). A German emperor, possibly Staufer Frederick II, was interested in languages and initiated a tragic experiment. In order to find out which language children would speak if they were not exposed to any language, he forbade the staff in an orphanage to speak to the young children in their care. The experiment ended tragically: not only did the children lack the ability to speak, but they also died because were deprived of affection as well as language.

Warmth and nutrition are visible and measurable; love and affection are not. A lack of nutrients can lead, for example, to impaired bone growth. This can also be seen or measured. A lack of love and affection may not be visible, but it still leads to a restriction of emotional and mental growth. The unfolding of the personality requires trust, preferably basic or primal trust. The treatment state in Shiatsu opens the door to trust and thus to a deep and positive experience that is often lost. More than once I have experienced how the rediscovery of trust has spontaneously triggered emotional growth processes, and made up for developments that could not take place in childhood and adolescence. It is important to note that this is not primarily a trust in the person of the practitioner or guide, but a trust that arises within the client and can be accessed independently of other individuals. A comforting »trust in the earth« can be a first step in this direction. The basic feeling of »I have to carry myself« slowly develops into a feeling of »I am being carried«.

If our client has been able to follow us up to this point, they are now reasonably relaxed, grounded, collected, centred, alert and calm. With the next sentence:

»At the end, take a moment to feel within yourself once again and see how you are, how you perceive yourself«,

we gently guide them into contact with their overall condition, which also includes their emotional state. Neurobiologists have found that even our basic mood, whether we feel good, average or bad, is composed of subtle body signals. We have already learned that we can influence internal processes when we learn to perceive them. If we don't notice our bad posture, we can hardly do anything about it. Biofeedback studies show that most people can learn to slow down or speed up their heartbeat in a short time, if they are aware of it, for example, by being made to hear it via loudspeakers. Similarly, many migraine patients are able to reduce tension in blood vessels leading to the head when their state of tension is made visible or audible using technical devices. In the more recently developed neurofeedback, people even learn to harmonise their EEG. They see an airplane on a screen and are asked to make it land. When their EEG harmonizes and moves in the right direction, the plane begins the descent for landing, and when it gets more chaotic, it ascends. They can't explain how they do it, but the fact is that they can. Unlike individual physiological functions such as heartbeat or blood vessel tension, listening to our inner body space, to our body field, fundamentally includes all physiological and psycho-spiritual processes, since on the level of the body field, there is no separation between body, mind and soul.

Listening to one's own body plays a central role in Focusing as developed by Eugene Gendlin. For him, Focusing means watching life take its next developmental step. Also in Shiatsu, opportunities can arise for the client to become aware of life force in their process of unfolding and thus to meet their true teacher, life itself.

The last sentence of our guided attunement is:

»At the end of the treatment, you will have another opportunity to feel inside yourself and compare your experience with the current one. You can use the treatment to feel yourself in every touch, every point and every moment.«

Through this pre-Shiatsu attunement, the client is shown that their experience and the relationship with themselves are at the centre of attention. The treatment is merely a means to better and perhaps more deeply understand oneself and find the way out of self-alienation and into self-contact. It fosters curiosity about what is to come and serves as an aid to staying present and focused on oneself. One difficulty that often arises at this point is that some people may be reluctant to look at or even feel something uncomfortable within themselves. The suggestion that there will be an opportunity at the end of the treatment to consciously turn to one's own inner experience and compare it with the initial experience not only gives hope that something might change through the subsequent Shiatsu treatment, but also helps to open up to the uncomfortable aspects of the present. After all, in order to really compare, one must have perceived the initial experience with clarity.

Many Shiatsu practitioners avoid speaking during the treatment, as silence is one of the essential factors for the effectiveness of Shiatsu. I myself studied Shiatsu from 1979 to 1981 with Shizuto Masunaga at the IOKAI in Tokyo. There, four to six practitioners treated their clients at the same time in one room, there was a lot of talking and sometime laughing, and at times it was quiet again. It was not until I returned to Germany and started practicing Qigong more intensively that I realised that the Japanese, and other Asian people perceive the world and their fellow human beings more through their body field than with our familiar five senses. This kind of perception or attunement, which we have unfortunately lost to a great extent, makes it possible to speak and still remain in sensitive contact with the treatment process. There is even a specific term in Japanese for this process of spreading one's Ki in space: *kehai*. That which the Japanese still have as cultural heritage, is something we often have to work hard to acquire.

Nevertheless, silence and stillness have a quality of their own that is worth honouring. If you are used to this and wish to continue, it makes sense to resume verbal communication only at the end of the treatment. However, it can also be helpful to ask questions in between to help focus the client's attention on specific inner perceptions, thereby increasing their effectiveness. For example, after treating a leg, we can invite the client to feel their legs and notice any differences, or if we feel an energy flow, we can ask them about their internal experience to bring this nourishing occurrence into their field of attention. There are many ways to communicate during the treatment and thereby increase the client's self-awareness. At the end of the treatment, we can ask the client once again about their inner experience with the following words:

»Keep your eyes closed, remain in the state you are in, feel inside yourself again, and express in a few words how you feel and what has changed.«

It is important that the client is still in the treatment state, so that they can search for the right words from the presence of their experience. Often, the description begins with the words »it's really hard to put into words«. This is an excellent sign that the client is in contact with an experience that is beyond words and therefore beyond conscious understanding. Their waking consciousness, in which they communicate with us, comes into contact with a wealth of previously unconscious body signals. Ultimately, it's not important whether they find the exact words; what is important is the attempt, for to find words for something is to become aware of the event for which words are sought. This is the beginning of an inner adventure.

This reference to one's own inner experience seems to me to be important when we want to treat a client according to the principles of Traditional Chinese Medicine (TCM). A few years ago, I worked closely with a doctor who treated his patients, with Mora therapy, an advanced form of electro-acupuncture. In this method a metal probe measures the skin resistance at the beginning and end points of the meridians on the fingertips and toes, and the readings are projected onto a screen. We wanted to see if the changes induced by Shiatsu treatments could be measured in this way.

A mutual patient volunteered for our experiment. We started by having the doctor measure the patient's data. To his surprise, the readings were all around the normal average. Usually, there are deviations up or down in various meridians, rather like Kyō and Jitsu. These are then treated with the aim of restoring balance, so in this case, we were unsure of what to do, since a Shiatsu treatment could not have improved the result.

Somehow, we got talking, and I asked the patient – without any conscious therapeutic reference – how she was feeling. She began to talk about a bus trip to Turkey from which she had just returned and became more and more excited. It turned out that she had on the trip gained distance from her marital problems – her husband was having an affair – or more precisely, had run away from them. When she finally got on the bus, thinking she could leave everything behind, at least for a while, she struck up a conversation with the person sitting next to her and it turned out that this person knew her husband. Her dream of running away had been shattered, and all the problems with her husband essentially travelled with her on the bus to Turkey.

By the time she had arrived at the doctor's practice for our little experiment, she had forgotten all about it and was fine. Now that she was talking about it, all the anger and frustration about her husband overwhelmed her all over again. I suggested to the doctor that we take another reading, and lo and behold, the data associated with the gallbladder meridian had plummeted (however that is to be judged energetically). I concluded that the state of a meridian system, or what can be measured in this way, depends on whether a specific issue or problem is activated or repressed, forgotten or put aside, meaning that we are successfully taking a break from it.

This raises the question of how far a Shiatsu treatment, which is part of a holiday from everyday life and energy-sapping problems, and is indeed part of this distancing, can really help to cope with daily challenges. When we ask our clients about a specific issue at the beginning of a session, they have the opportunity to consciously bring any difficulties they are facing into the session or leave them aside. Their conscious self then makes the decision. However, it is not uncommon for the silence and sensibility inherent in a Shiatsu treatment to reveal what has been suppressed and pushed away but is pressing into life with great force, and needs to be looked at and resolved. In this case, the person's soul, striving for wholeness, seems to want to determine the course of events more than the conscious ego. This tension between the natural urge of the soul to resolve and repression by the ego is often the background to energetic blockages and thus all kinds of physical and psychological disorders. Without knowing the specifics of the background, what our hands perceive as hardness, congestion, lifelessness, coldness, kyō or jitsu are the consequences of this tension. The onset of the flow of life force, a pleasant warmth and relaxation, the experience of expansiveness and wholeness, indicate the dissolution of the field of tension and the integration of forces that the client – consciously or unconsciously – did not want to give space to in their life before.

To summarise, our personal issues, whether consciously brought into the treatment or brought up from the unconscious, can have a significant impact on the energy levels in our meridians and our entire energy system. Through the sensitive perception of the inner space, the client comes into contact with these issues without having to specify or name them individually. The Shiatsu practitioner's art of treatment is thus complemented by the client's growing art of living, for it can truly be described as an art of living when someone manages to live with their issues rather than against them.

Returning to our verbal guidance, if, in response to our question, our client has perceived differences between the state at the beginning and at the end of the treatment, they may still not automatically understand what that means for them and their life. When we ask them – still with their eyes closed – what would be different in their life or in specific situations of their life if what they are experiencing now was always available to them, we make a connection between the treatment experience and the client's everyday life. Since all of this happens in the treatment state, the impact is deeper and more lasting than it would be if we did this in a conversation after the treatment. The client can get an idea, from their own experience, of the kind of support that Shiatsu can provide. It is helpful to remember this final impression of the client or to write in down using keywords, so that we can pick up the thread at the beginning of the next treatment, for example with the question: »How have you been feeling since the last session? How long did you feel the lightness and inner expansiveness, and how has it affected your life?«

Although there are typical and relatively common descriptions, it is always a highly individual experience. The client understands that it is all about them personally and that they are being given a tool to influence their life. This becomes even clearer when we give them a little homework: to lie down at home, close their eyes, and recall and reactivate the Shiatsu experience. Some clients manage this from the beginning and most learn within a few sessions. With this experience, the client becomes aware that their experience may have been initiated with the help of a Shiatsu practitioner at the beginning, but ultimately does not depend on the practitioner. The client learns to independently access a nourishing, organising and transforming process. The work is not done by them – just as little as by his companion – the work is done by the ki, their very life force. They simply learn to create the internal atmosphere it requires to become active.

Let's summarise what has been said so far: While a practitioner is more like a taxi driver, who takes a passenger to a certain destination (e.g., pain relief) without the passenger having to do anything – apart from paying – a companion works as a driving instructor, with the aim of not only showing the way but also teaching the passenger how to drive the car. The most important tool in this process is the training of attention, through which the client learns to relate to their own inner experiences. In this awareness, body, mind, and soul naturally become one.

The guided attunement at the beginning of the treatment can also be continued and further developed by the client as an independent exercise. The attunement, initially enunciated by the companion, can be carried out by the client in a ritualised form, similar to autogenic training. However, they will still need competent guidance regarding what they experience during the exercise. The focus of the exercise is in the mental and energetic realm, i.e., it is less about the *what* and more about the *how*. It is primarily about training the ability to centre oneself and to become aware of energetic processes. Exercises with this focus have a more subtle and deeper effect than, for example, physical exercises, which are also beneficial for the mind and soul, but may not achieve the same intensity and depth.

The training of attention, as described here, and Shiatsu complement and support each other. The treatment becomes an exercise for the client, and the experience of the treatment can be incorporated into their own practice by updating it with the help of their memory. The energy body experience that develops in this way is life experience in the most direct sense. As life unfolds within a person, the person unfolds within life.

5

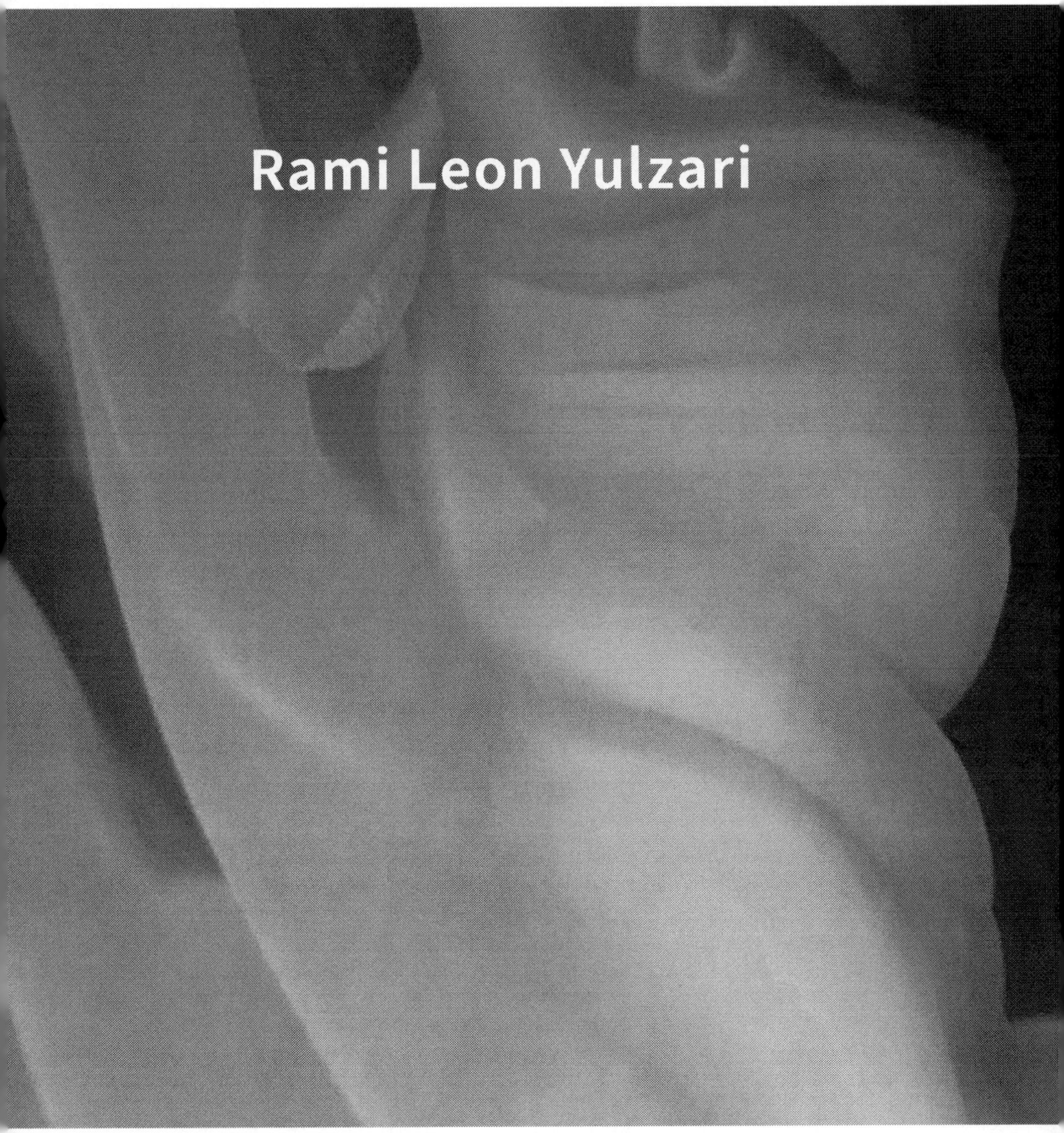

Rami Leon Yulzari

Pictures in a Treatment Room

” The hand cannot touch itself and the eye cannot see itself. I touch the hand and look into the eye, and yet the hand cannot touch itself and the eye cannot see itself. It is possible to rest on waves that have unknown depths beneath them, to close one‘s eyes to the sun that will soon sink.

1.

She was wearing a dark brown T-shirt and a green, almost turquoise shirt. Over these she wore a puffy, sleeveless coat of faded purple that resembled a soldier‘s vest. She was wiping away tears with the back of her hand, and her cheekbones turned to red stains. I travelled with Matisse in Morocco. When I came back from wandering and looked into her eyes, she took off her vest. So it happened. I was able then to wrap her head in my hands.

2.

I watched her white hand lying limply on a sheet of faded blue. The skin on the back of the hand was smooth and soft, not showing the blue marks of blood vessels or the redness of skin disease, a limp palm lacking the signs of life that mark other parts of the body. Like the hand of the Madonna, against the blue of her dress, reaching out to her child and not touching it.

3.

He sits across from me, his back arched and his chin tilted forward, accentuating the thinness of his throat and the bulge of his Adam's apple, where hairs remain after a not very careful shave, of someone who has lost his patience while shaving and he says to himself, for what and for whom, who will look at my throat and whoever will look, I want him to love me with the hairs on my throat and he or she would love me so much that the little hairs on my Adam's apple would disappear as if they had never been there.

4.

She jumped abruptly, with a quick, sharp movement. At once, she moved from lying to sitting and looked at me with eyes that do not see, that have nothing from life and nothing from her life is reflected in them. I could not get close to her and I could not get away from her, and so we stayed just at this exact distance that was immobile, motionless and almost breathless for a very long time, until she was aware of the dryness of her lips.

5.

His hair is abundant despite his age. Whenever he imagines that his hair is not in order, he slips it gently and puts it back in place, because the hair has to be in order, it is what closes his head from above and does not allow his ceaseless thoughts, the sound of squeaking and screeching voices and the sound of birds flying in panic, dissolve into the gaping space above him. He knows that the thoughts are fluttering in their cage that is his head and if only, and even for a moment, the hair will not be in place, they will flutter in all directions and the body they leave will be emptied and its contents will drain into the spaces even the smallest on the surface beneath his feet no matter where he will be and on what he will stand or sit or lie, everything that has a space in it and into it he will fade away.

6.

More than by the wrinkles, her age is revealed by an involuntary movement of the jaw, a kind of rearrangement of the mouth, reminiscent of false teeth. When I hold her hand, she clenches her fingers around my thumb in a baby reflex. Whenever she does this, the movement of her mouth seems to be a nursing reflex. An old woman and a baby, a baby and an old woman.

7.

I saw his head as that of an eagle, resting on a thin, crooked neck. I remembered that eagles feed on carcasses, and that all their strength and the size of their wings and their amazing gliding is over carcasses, and I thought that the old man was nourished by his memories, and with him, miraculously, the carcasses do not disappear, but grow and swell, and one day, and perhaps very soon, they will swell so much that they will envelop him, and he will live in his memories and not on them.

8.

It was raining or not, in the room we both heard its voice. Light clouds covered the ceiling and filtered the light that became softer, blurring the features of your face that were melting into small puddles formed around us. I dipped my fingers in them. The water trickled into my hands which were covering your eyes and revived memories of youth, the sight of rain falling unceasingly on the sea. You were touched by water from heaven and water from the sea. It had the sound of water touching fire, the fire of emotions overflowing the heart, scorching the inside of the body, drying the respiratory passages and waking you up before dawn choking, breathless, with eyes wide open to see what is not to be seen. It was raining or not. The bougainvillea had the look of a bougainvillea, the rosemary smelled of rosemary.

9.

When I move, there is movement in her body. Her head turns to me even with her eyes closed, like a sunflower leaning towards the sun. Her heart beats in her throat, my heart beats in my throat. The sun is in the sky I talk to myself, it shines and sinks, sinks and shines. I adjust my breath to her breath, we inhale and exhale together.

10.

She is lying on the bed from which she will not get up again. I sit beside her. Next to her head, a moth clings to a wall from which it will not fly. I look alternately at her face and at the moth. I wonder at the sound of the inhalation machine that does not distinguish between inhalation and exhalation. From time to time I check to see if she is still breathing. From time to time I think whether the moth is still alive. Life and death are one? Certainly not two. Her hand between my two palms.

11.

When she could no longer bear the sound of thunder rising from the inside of her brain, a noise created by collisions between the clouds of thoughts and clouds of emotion, rolling up into the meninges and creating unbearable pain as it tries to break through the dome of the skull, she dropped herself like from a high cliff, to the knee beside her, presses the center of the chest to the hard bone with the force of someone who clings to what cannot be separated from it.

12.

I heard the vibration in her voice, like the sound of a flapping wing shaking the air before landing. The palm of my hand adapted to the socket on her shoulder and the other to the shoulder blade mound, and together they held a small trembling bird until she calmed down. You could not be sure when the noise had stopped. You could hear it fading away, becoming a distant memory as her breathing slowed and deepened. For a long time, she wobbled exhausted on the edge of sleep until she fell asleep.

13.

I listen to her breathing, accompanied by the squeaky sound of air being blocked. I place my hand on her chest and her breath is a muffled sound rising from the depths. When I raise my hand, a heavy, heartbreaking sigh comes from the dim depths of her memory.

14.

»Where's my pillow?« asked the elderly woman in a baby voice. Where's my pillow? Mine? Mine? When I put the pillow to her head, her head fell on it. She buried herself in it, inhaling its scent. Slowly it grew dark, and very slowly she removed her limbs, her arms and legs, her shoulders, and her heart widened to her dreams.

15.

When her palm rests on my palm and my thumb touches the center of her palm, her thumb moves in my hand like an uvula, oscillating and tapping the bell of the skin between my fingers, sending sounds that echo all the way to my heart, somewhere in the unfathomable space between two people.

16.

I could see the movement of the tendons in the neck every time the jaw moved, a movement of skin that was no longer the tense movement of time passing. The jaw moved and moved because she spoke and spoke and her words rose up on her face, above her head, and gathered around her head like a telescope of distant stars, where material produced by explosions and flares and collisions became lumps of thick clouds moving in circular orbits around stars or black holes not yet seen.

17.

I lean against what connects and separates us, compressing it until it becomes almost solid. It is hard and airy at the same time, like an inflated rubber ball. If you push it, it pushes back. I lean and it pushes until the movement is small and slow and quiet and we lean on each other and we do not have to carry our weight and the weight of our thoughts and the weight of our feelings. The movement of the pendulum has stopped.

18.

I hear her voice speaking to me. At the same time, I hear the daughter of her voice talking to herself. I hear her voice and the daughter of my hearing hears the daughter of her voice and together they all spin and whirl like a flock of swifts and like them do not land and do not rest as they fly.

19.

When I move and stop touching her, she rises as if in sleep, with the slow movements of someone who has rediscovered the possibility of movement. She seems to return from a deep, dark night to a blinding midday light. She looks up and meets her reflection. I let her look out of my eyes. She looks so exposed, so vulnerable. I go back to her and hug her shoulders until her gaze brightens, her back stabilises and her face rises.

20.

The light outside is descending and the light within has not yet risen, something is about to be revealed. There is a hint in the smell of jasmine. I can feel the vibrating feathers of a newly hatched chick touching the inside of my palms, covering her eyes like two bowls. A wave of vibration runs through her whole body, my whole body. The wind is quiet.

Pieta

And these are her bodily fluids, collected in the palms of my hands that cover her face: the sweat from her forehead, the tears that would not stop, the snot dripping from her nose, the blood pouring incessantly from her nostrils into my fingers. The blood, poured into the transparent liquids, weaves in thin embroidery threads the watery shroud that envelops her child.

1.

She is lying on her back. I sit beside her. Her face is soft, her eyelids peaceful, like Ophelia's face floating in the river. I put the palm of my hand on her forehead and her forehead fills my palm. I smooth the wrinkles on her forehead, put a finger on her third eye, searching for the fourth, the fifth.

2.

When I touch her belly, she remembers them, her son and his son, who died together. Then a crescent moon whitened on her cheek, and its rays illuminate the ladder that is placed on earth, and its head touch heaven, on which her son and his son go up and down.

3.

I hold the arm straight, letting the forearm slowly open. A sigh is born, rolling from the depth of the chest to the shoulder socket, from there to the arm and emanating from the center of her palm. I am listening.

4.

His head is between my palms, one supporting his neck and the other covering his forehead. I wait until his thoughts slow down and his head becomes heavy. I remember Zeus, whose daughter was born from his head. The unbearable pain in his neck, I think, are the contractions for the rebirth of his dead daughter.

5.

My fingers wander on the head, in an unknown land under the hair, climbing mountains, sliding down the slopes, painting the map of the new land. They are attentive to the echoes that rise from the ravines. The fontanel is a wide valley and its sound is deep and slow. From there, suddenly, rises a bleat of the baby he is, lying on his back, his eyes open and all his limbs moving in harmony.

6.

I touch the bulging bone at the back of the head, listening to broadcasts. What do you hear? I ask you, what do you hear? You hear yourself, the sounds of the intestines, the pounding of blood, you hear life and all the rest is the incessant murmur of your mind.

7.

When my daughter died, she said, a cloud passed over the sun and we both covered ourselves with shadow. Since then, the movement of my life is a movement of longing, the loop of blood flowing from my heart to my heart. Touching the pulse, sinking into the space between the heartbeats, there I am with my daughter in my arms. What I have seen floats in the fluid of my eyes, what I have felt sinks to the bottom of my heart. What floats will sink and what has sunk is a continuous present.

8.

She shows me a photograph of her daughter, moments after her death, when she is as beautiful as an angel. When she cries, a smell of earth after rain comes to my nose. What I cannot contain, I breathe out; what trembles my heart, I breathe in.

9.

I look at her from my eyes. She bows her head. When she looks up, looks at her through my eyes, she sees possibilities: to pick up a trampled autumn crocus, to accompany an ant on its journey, to watch a slow sunset through the pine trees lace.

10.

The hand cannot touch itself and the eye cannot see itself. I touch the hand and look into the eye, and yet the hand cannot touch itself and the eye cannot see itself. It is possible to rest on waves that have unknown depths beneath them, to close one‘s eyes to the sun that will soon sink.

6

Chris McAlister

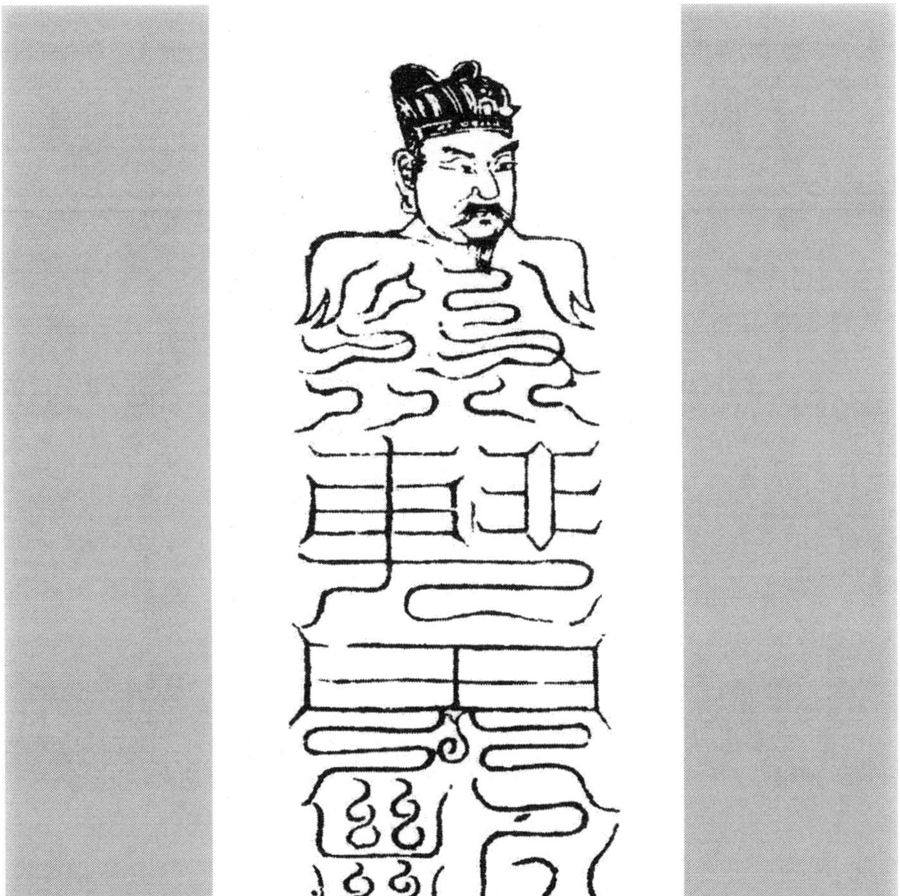

The Alchemy of Words

”Even the most rational and logically cemented person can enter the world of imagery when the name of an acupoint is mentioned. They will, of course, have their own personal and completely individual associations to the images evoked – all the more reason to use them.

Non-verbal Communication

Just like all touch-based practices, Shiatsu involves a high level of non-verbal communication.

Indeed, in the East it is fairly often practised in near total silence. This probably relates to the way Oriental people tend to somatise emotional and spiritual issues. For example, my acupuncture teacher almost exclusively treated lower back, neck and knee problems, and though he would talk to his patients and even joke around with them, there were never any in-depth conversations about aspects of the soul.

It is therefore no great surprise that psychoanalysis and all of its offspring and offshoots trace their origins to Europe. The value of verbal communication in therapy received a formal recognition and the world was never the same again. On the other hand, there are far older traditions when it comes to verbal communication in the Western world, foremost among them, perhaps, storytelling.

Storytelling

Long before the age of letters and printing, news was spread and history was preserved through the spoken word. The art of storytelling was based on several abilities, one of them of course being memory – the teller would need an enormous capacity for memorisation to maintain the store of tales to be told and handed down.

Other useful skills would probably have included cadence – the ability to raise and lower the tone and intensity of voice to create tension or space. Imagery and descriptive elements would likewise have been vital tools, as would the ability to pace – some sections would be sped through almost without pause, while others would need to be recounted very slowly, to allow the import to truly shine and sink deeply into the listeners' consciousness. Even pure silence would likely have been a vital tool – to be used sagely, when required.

A truly vital element of all storytelling is imagery. If a picture paints a thousand words, then how potent are poetic images skillfully used by master storytellers? An image travels instantly into the very heart, the mind's eye of the listener. It evokes wholly unique pictures from the realms of imagination and from the depths of memory – both the personal memory of the individual and the ancestral memories stored in the communal banks of family, tribe and nation.

At the end of the formal telling, it is likely that there arose spontaneous discussions, questions, answers, alternative versions proposed, deeper analysis of certain elements and above all a time for ventilation, both individually and in group format. Naturally, certain gifted individuals would give voice to the memories and images that surfaced from within them during the story and share them for the enrichment of the group. In this way the story was almost certainly tweaked and honed over the generations of its telling.

All of the tools and features mentioned above can be extremely useful during our Shiatsu sessions. Needless to say, each client, and indeed each and every treatment session will require its own proportions of these elements, and constant attention is required to adapt and modify the flow of the treatment as it develops. No two are ever the same and no formula can cover the eventualities this entails.

A Wonderful Vocabulary

Oriental medicine provides a wonderful vocabulary for the telling of stories. Each acupoint has a more or less intriguing and mysterious name. Every concept, be it Shen, Qi, Jing, Ling or Wind evokes images that open mental and spiritual vistas in both giver and receiver. These can be used, when appropriate, to deepen or broaden the effects of our touch, pressure and opening techniques.

The opposite is also true of course, for at times our clients will relate stories of things they have experienced in their lives, in their dreams or even in the visions catalysed by Shiatsu itself. Such times can be wonderful learning opportunities for us as Shiatsu givers, as we recall that the main reason for our practice is ultimately our own development – both for ourselves and for the people and the world around us.

Optimally then, storytelling comes from both sides of the relationship, each having the opportunity to find their world enriched by the other. Recently I was involved in a situation where these gifts were shared in a stunning joint learning experience.

Working on What has been Spoiled

Gloria had visited me previously for a series of treatments and had recently returned. This was to be our second session, following a harrowing experience at the hands of an anaesiology unit at the local university hospital. After long deliberation, she had gone against her gut feeling and submitted to a gastroscopic examination with full anaesthetic. When she regained consciousness, she was distressed to realise that her jaw had been dislocated, resulting in immense pain and shooting tinnitus.

She had consulted a chiropractor, who had helped her reset the mechanics of the jaw joint but was still experiencing extreme muscular pain and multi-tonal ringing in the ears. In addition, it had been confirmed that her throat was badly injured from the intubation. She was not at all a happy camper as we met for our second session.

After some preliminary work to relax her on a general level, I moved up to the head and neck area to see what might be done about the tinnitus from a local perspective. Having worked with some of the meridians flowing through the neck, I asked her where she was experiencing the tinnitus at that precise moment. To both my and her own surprise, she responded that it was mainly in the outer portion of the ear, rather than deep inside the inner ear.

I asked her to guide me as I very gently placed my fingers close to her ear. She guided me towards the earlobe and then, very slowly and very gradually, into the lower, inner portion of her ear. We were lightheartedly swopping information and ideas all the way and, it seemed to me, getting closer and closer to some kind of epicentrum, when suddenly she shook my hands away and told me in no uncertain terms that this was not working and that she could not possibly guide me any further.

Maximum Space

I was, to say the least, very surprised. Gloria and I had been on easy terms since the very first time I met her and seemed to have a very clear understanding of how our dialogue and cooperation was progressing. I backed off, feeling somewhat confused, and assumed a new position, nearer her feet to give her maximum space, while still remaining in physical contact. She seemed unable to communicate at first and I found myself very quietly awaiting what might happen from here.

What happened was that she began to speak, in a hesitant and uncertain way. She seemed to be groping for some kind of understanding as to what had just happened. After a short while, she asked whether I was upset, to which I responded that no, I was not upset but somewhat confused. She nodded slightly, seeming to understand. A short silence followed, in which she seemed to continue working through her responses. She then apologised to me, which I certainly had not expected. I told her there was absolutely no need to apologise, but that I was as keen as she to understand what had transpired in that momentary explosion.

She seemed to retreat inside again, and after a short while returned with a partial explanation. The presence of my fingers inside her outer ear, together with the casual way I was conversing with her had set something off; something irrational. This was related to her vulnerability and, to use her own words, the carelessness she had perceived in the attitude of the anaesthiologist and his team. Suddenly, she had imagined them laughing and joking in an irreverent fashion over her inert and helpless body.

To add to this feeling of external insult, she realised that she was harbouring shame over the way she had forced her body into undergoing this procedure, which she knew she did not want to experience. She started to cry, expressing sorrow verbally through her tears, over the betrayal she had enacted on her body. I suggested she might simply apologise to her body, which she immediately began to do, and with this a slight softening of her voice and posture became apparent.

It was here the real change started.

Missing Parts

She began, very hesitantly, to describe her state of mind as she regained consciousness after the procedure at the hospital. Not quite understanding it herself, she explained that it had felt as though a part of her was missing – an important part – that she felt incomplete, partial, lacking in some significant sense. This was no surprise for me and I immediately set to work on the point at the very top of her head, GV 20, the Hundred Meetings. Not only is this said to be a point where all the meridians (roughly one hundred in total) come together; it is also a point well known in several traditions, including the Chinese one, for reuniting parts of the spirit lost after traumatic experiences: soul retrieval.

She was softly crying, still vaguely apologetic towards her body for what she had exposed it to, as I then moved to her upper back and the points on the outer Bladder meridian. There is a series of points interspersed along this meridian, which I and many others know as the Spirit points. They are named after the five psycho-spiritual aspects of the

Oriental energy system: Po, Shen, Hun, Yi and Zhi. These correspond to the energies of the five elements and the points themselves create a kind of horizontal line that includes the relevant Shu point and the Du Mai point in the centre. Energy bands that run horizontally across the body are thus created, giving one the possibility to work to and fro across the spine within the zone thus formed.

Spirit Points

I began with the the points just outside the Lung Shu points, those corresponding to the psychological energy of Metal: Po He, the doors of the Po. The Po is known as the animal or corporeal spirit, meaning that it guards the body's integrity in a more or less instinctual way. Her crying increased slightly in both volume and intensity. This was wholly unsurprising. The Po had received a grievous insult with the decision to undergo a procedure, which she knew through her internal body sense that she did not want to experience.

Then we moved down two points.

The next points I settled into were the ones situated just outside the Heart Shu points. They are called Shen Tang, and while Shen is usually translated as spirit, Tang means hall. What I believe is meant here is a special kind of room, one that is finer in all its attributes and worthy of the Emperor (or Empress!) I noticed another increase in intensity and by now her crying had become a kind of racking, shaking, whole body phenomenon.

I explained very gently and very slowly where we were and the symbolism inherent in the name of the points. Speaking slowly, I was able to calm her and gain her listening attention. Choosing my words with great care, I described how this special room might look. Knowing Gloria for a person with a highly developed aesthetic sense, I believed I could engage her in this description. Indeed, it seemed to be working, as her crying began to soften and slow.

I took time to describe the various attributes of how this hall might look, including such features as curtains, wall hangings, candelabras, windows and furniture – all of the finest quality and of the most wondrous appearance. She nodded from time to time but maintained complete silence as I spoke. When I had said all I wanted to and the crying had completely finished, I asked her whether she had been able to create her own spirit hall and if so what it looked like. I fully expected some version of the image I had described for her.

Imagine my surprise when her spirit hall was utterly unlike the image I had created. She spoke very softly and very slowly as she told me the where and the how of her special place.

A Very Special Place

First of all, it was outdoors. That was my first surprise. She was seated with her back against a large tree and felt completely secure. She was in some a kind of field and the grass beneath her was soft and dry. Before her was a fire – the fire was warm and comforting. Anyone who knows anything about the five elements will already have grasped my second major surprise here. The Shen is said to belong to the Fire element, but I had not mentioned this feature, deeming it a potentially complicating and otherwise irrelevant factor in the process. She had found it all by herself.

There was a feeling of her being in the presence of nature's most comforting forces and feeling entirely at ease. Very soon after this, I felt able to round off the session and left her in the room for a few minutes alone, as is my custom. She emerged a few minutes later and went to sit with her mother in another room, where I left them in peace to communicate with each other, while I fixed tea for them both in the kitchen – within earshot but unable to hear the details of their conversation. A few minutes later, Gloria came into the kitchen and looked at me wide-eyed and widely smiling.

Next time she came, one week later, we were back on track in a fundamental way. The muscular pains were only slightly relieved and the tinnitus only partially diminished, but her whole manner was different. She was herself again in a sense that gave her the confidence to grasp and proceed with her healing process.

Exact Coordinates

Reflecting on this experience, I draw several conclusions.

Firstly, this experience would have been extremely difficult to generate without the use of verbal communication. Without being able to receive exact coordinates for Gloria's emotional, energetic and spiritual whereabouts, I would not have been led to the points and descriptions I used.

Without my prompts and clues, her experience of trauma would have remained deeply frozen within her and her Shen experience would have remained inaccessible and thus purely hypothetical.

Secondly, it confirmed the rich magic inherent in the language of Oriental medicine and the value of using it, sparingly, in the treatment context. This fathomless vein of infinite wealth is a resource that I feel is often neglected in our modern version of the ancient tradition. Even the most rational and logically cemented person can enter the world of imagery when the name of an acupoint is mentioned. They will, of course, have their own personal and completely individual associations to the images evoked – all the more reason to use them.

Thirdly, it reconfirmed for me the enormous power a client can retrieve when they are given the tools – and the space – to tell their own story. In their own words. It is a source of enormous personal power to be given time and space and support to investigate one's own narrative. Many people, on entering our world of Shiatsu and Oriental medicine, find multiple access to avenues long blocked within their own labyrinth of experience. A part of the richness of our work as practitioners and facilitators lies in the witnessing of these unique and unexpected tales from within.

7

Chris McAlister

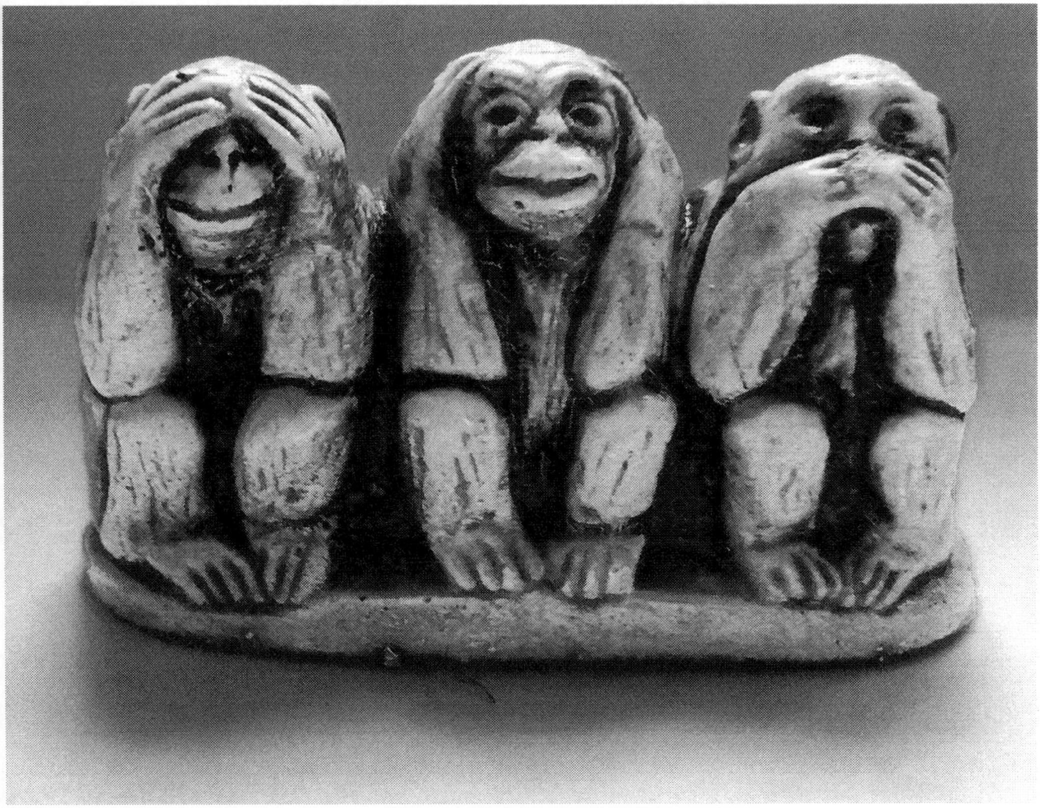

To Speak or Not to Speak?

But also:

When and How to Speak?
Those are the Questions!

”

Jokes and humour have become a key part of my interaction with clients, levity being the antidote to tension – Shakespeare, for example, was well aware of this and made a point in several of his dramas of having a »fool« outline painful or embarrassing truths for noble men, who’s minds had skillfully managed to evade said truths.

My main Shiatsu teacher in Japan, Takeo Suzuki, was what I have come to view as an eccentric genius. His tactile intelligence, his intuitive connection with life force-energy and his ability to interact with it in a wholly devoted, focused and detailed manner is something I have yet to see surpassed: genius. His almost complete lack of interest in social interaction, his sheer single-mindedness and his almost total lack of communication skills are what lead me to use the word »eccentric«.

In the three years I attended his weekly classes (all day, every Monday!) I learned absolutely zero about his private person other than the fact that he, at some point, had practiced judo, that he used swimming as his primary physical Qi research forum and that he enjoyed watching television as a matrix for interaction with Qi in various fields.

An example of the latter was provided when he explained on a given Monday morning that he had received specific information regarding the various functions of the meridians with respect to the anatomy and physiology of the eye ... while watching television.

He even invented a series of exercises for the perception and release of life force energy while watching a TV programme on Taiji and Qigong. Needless to say, the movements he invented – and unleashed on a bewildered but fascinated set of pupils – were not only genial in their simplicity but pure eccentricity in their aesthetic apparel. To this day, I still smile while doing them.

The limits of his communicative skills lay purely on the verbal and social levels. In sharp contrast, he could communicate directly through energy transmission with plants and with people thousands of miles way – energetically, not through words.

A typical treatment with him was initiated through a polite enquiry as to the state of play regarding the subject's health. This was dispensed with as summarily as possible, so that the real work of energetic communication could start without unnecessary delay. This work was then diligently pursued for approximately 55 minutes, at which point the subject was carefully covered with a blanket. Suzuki would then swiftly and smoothly remove himself to a similar futon several metres away to start the next treatment. (He had seven or eight futons lined up, from which one was at liberty to choose).

The idea – verbally unexpressed – was that the subject would at some – verbally unspecified – point in time place the money payable for said treatment somewhere visible, while bowing, which would occasion a slight bowing of the head and an immediate return to energetic work with the current subject.

Suzuki was one of Masunaga's later students. According to one of the senior students in the class, he was asked by Masunaga to treat him, as the latter realised the extent of his sickness towards the end of his life – not an insignificant honour, perhaps.

Suzuki's personal mission seems to have been to develop and simplify the work of his teacher. He went to some lengths to simplify the katas he himself had learnt and instead focused on the quality of the pressure, working from and considerably refining Masunaga's principles of natural pressure.

Correspondingly, we spent hundreds of hours working with the simplest elements of Shiatsu: posture, pressure, relaxation and Qi perception. We also devoted many, many hours to the arcane subjects of meridian energetics and diagnosis. One subject we devoted precisely no hours at all to was verbal communication.

The consequence of all this?

I returned to Europe thoroughly drilled in all matters relating to posture, physical awareness and energy perception. This was, of course, an alloyed product of my combined training in Taiji chuan, acupuncture and Qigong. Nevertheless, in the vital sphere of conducting Shiatsu treatments with Western individuals, I swiftly found myself at an unexpected disadvantage.

A client who came for repeated treatments in the early days of my career as a therapist surprised me one day by remarking that I was unusually silent during and after treatments: »you never say anything« was more or less the gist of her comment. I was momentarily baffled, wondering what there was to say. The unspoken assumption underlying my Shiatsu training up to this point had been that the Qi did the work. My task, as therapist, was to interact with the Qi in as favourable, accurate and specific a way as possible. Beyond that the expectations placed upon me were almost non-existent.

Granted, there was the regrettable need to explain what Shiatsu (or acupuncture, or Taiji or Qigong) was to people with apparently no idea at all of what Qi was and how simple a matter it was to address it and work with it in a variety of ways. There was also the laborious necessity of designing flyers and information sheets describing the look, feel and benefits of all these surprisingly obscure activities to the same people. But surely, beyond that my task was crystal clear and free from doubt as to its outline and extent? Sadly not.

And so began my journey into verbal communication within the boundaries of Shiatsu treatments in a Western European country. I started by trying to explain what I was doing in terms of the linguistics of Oriental medicine, reasoning that if I could grasp it, then so could anyone else. Indeed, part of the lure of the practices I had so lovingly embraced was the very directness of this terminology with its wonderful, in-built imagery.

Needless to say, I was fully aware of the fundamental dictum: the Dao that can be explained in words is – of course! – not the true Dao. That went without saying. Mind cannot grasp the full extent or scope of reality – duh! But still and all, the poetic language devised, refined and nurtured through thousands of years of Oriental philosophical, spiritual and medical tradition was surely the key to the communication sought by these clients of mine.

Not.

Elaborate as well as simple descriptions of meridians, kyo and jitsu and the five elements failed – apparently and dismally – to electrify my clients as they had me in similar circumstances.

The situation was rendered even more farcical by the fact that my very first teachers in the Oriental tradition had not been able to communicate with me verbally at all. One reason for this was that my initial encounters took place in deepest South-Western China – not a place where English (or even French) was readily spoken in the mid 1980's. The other reason is that my first ever Shiatsu teacher was a deaf mute.

That is a long – and wonderful – story and one for another occasion, but very clearly fate had engineered my education in such a way as to eliminate the need for vast amounts of verbal explanation, leaving the way clear for bodily, energetic and intuitive communication to become the main instruments of transmission.

Since I therefore had no living examples to draw from, I was forced to make up my own method. Necessity being the mother of invention, I fell back on two sources of communication from earlier periods of my life: tomfoolery and the law. Strange bedfellows you'd think and rightly so, but not incompatible it transpires.

Taking these two in reverse order, my university legal education had taught me that water-tight logic is the only thing permitted in legal argumentation. Creative, even out of the box thinking, is certainly permitted but each level of your argument must rest unequivocally on the previous one. Statements must be brief and to the point. They must show direct connection and not waver from the line of reasoning.

Furthermore, and perhaps even more importantly, lines of questioning may not »lead«, it is said. You may not, by dint of questioning, lead the questionee into conclusions or even opinions based on your wish for a given outcome. You must therefore create the space for any outcome, including ones that you may not welcome.

This kind of communicative questioning, commonplace in psychotherapeutic circles, has recently come to be known as »neutral«, or »clean language« in various other therapeutic spheres, including Shiatsu. The important thing is that the therapist is not the creative impulse: the client is held and supported by questions that open spaces where insights, memories and images may arise spontaneously from within – uninfluenced by any goals, ambitions, blind spots or filters currently possessed by the therapist.

So much for the legal aspect of communicaton. Tomfoolery then? In a house with six children and an extended family of thirty cousins, the fool gains rapid access to a willing and enthusiastic audience. Combining spontaneously with any other wit or mimic present, the scene is set for a series of hilarious events, which certainly has its uses when it comes to lightening up mealtimes and family gatherings. The shift from family dynamics to the dynamics of the treatment room is not a huge one. Nor is it one of absoluteness, but simply one of degree.

Regarding both the requirements of legal questioning and the logistics of tomfoolery, the question is merely one of mindful modification and of judicious application.

In my own case, the final ingredient was curiosity. I am endlessly curious about what it is like to experience life as another person. Indeed, what causes anything to be as it is? How far back in the chain of causation can we reach to identify the various formative factors in any process? How do people cope with things? How does the body absorb psychic energy? How does a person manage their emotions?

These are questions that very clearly pertain to the dynamic equilibrium of health and ill health. But there are other intriguing questions that pop up spontaneously: languages, for example. Clients who speak, study or research languages are endlessly fascinating. Literature, to take another example. Clients who have any kind of literary appetite arouse my curiosity and thirst for knowledge. The list then stretches out: music, films, travel …

And that is before we have even touched on the big three: sex, religion and politics. Now, you may well argue – and you'd be right on the money – that these are somewhat touchy, not to say downright taboo subjects, especially in the treatment space – holy as it is. I would have to agree with you but calibrated with the dual instruments of legal process and tomfoolery, they become magical boxes that yield untold treasures.

There is no better way to get a feel for who you are dealing with than to allow someone to express themselves in one – or more – of these topical spheres. The key is not to engage personally. My opinions are almost worthless in this context – unless they are specifically elicited of course, and even then, need to be concisely rendered, focus immediately returning to the client themselves and their continued expression and development.

Jokes and humour have become a key part of my interaction with clients, levity being the antidote to tension – Shakespeare, for example, was well aware of this and made a point in several of his dramas of having a »fool« outline painful or embarrassing truths for noble men, who's minds had skillfully managed to evade said truths. At tense meetings, I have frequently witnessed the magical releasing effect of a joke spontaneously made – not at anyone's expense, but simply to remind the gathering that we all breathe and we all eat lunch and that maybe a short pause would help bring much needed oxygen to blood, brain and backside.

The mood, preoccupations and current concerns of that magical being, the client, are absolutely vital and wonderfully random factors in the communicative process. This is a veritable goldmine and one easily accessed. Let's face it: everyone likes talking about themselves; just more or less is the point. So, we need to be able to listen. Sounds simple, doesn't it? Well, it is simple; it's just not easy.

To truly listen is a skill that takes some learning for most of us. There is often that temptation to jump in and match the client's statement with one of your own, an opinion, an example, an elaboration, a negation … the list is endless. It really is a skill that requires much patience and many mistakes to develop. Most of us practise it with only partial success, and that is fine. Everything we do involves learning curves and listening is no exception. Listening may in fact, be one of the most difficult things we can engage in, given the fact that audial chatter is now a given constant in most modern milieu.

If we allow our clients to express themselves freely, they will, by doing so, effortlessly bring buried issues to the surface. At the very least, we will have given them the chance to ventilate and thereby expedite the process of relaxation by clearing space.

Our task then is to use the clean or neutral language of law and ethics to encourage them further: deeper into the most profound roots of trauma or upwards and outwards into the most exalted realms of the spirit.

Keep the joker card in your back pocket for use now and then, so things don't get too heavy.

8

Nick Pole

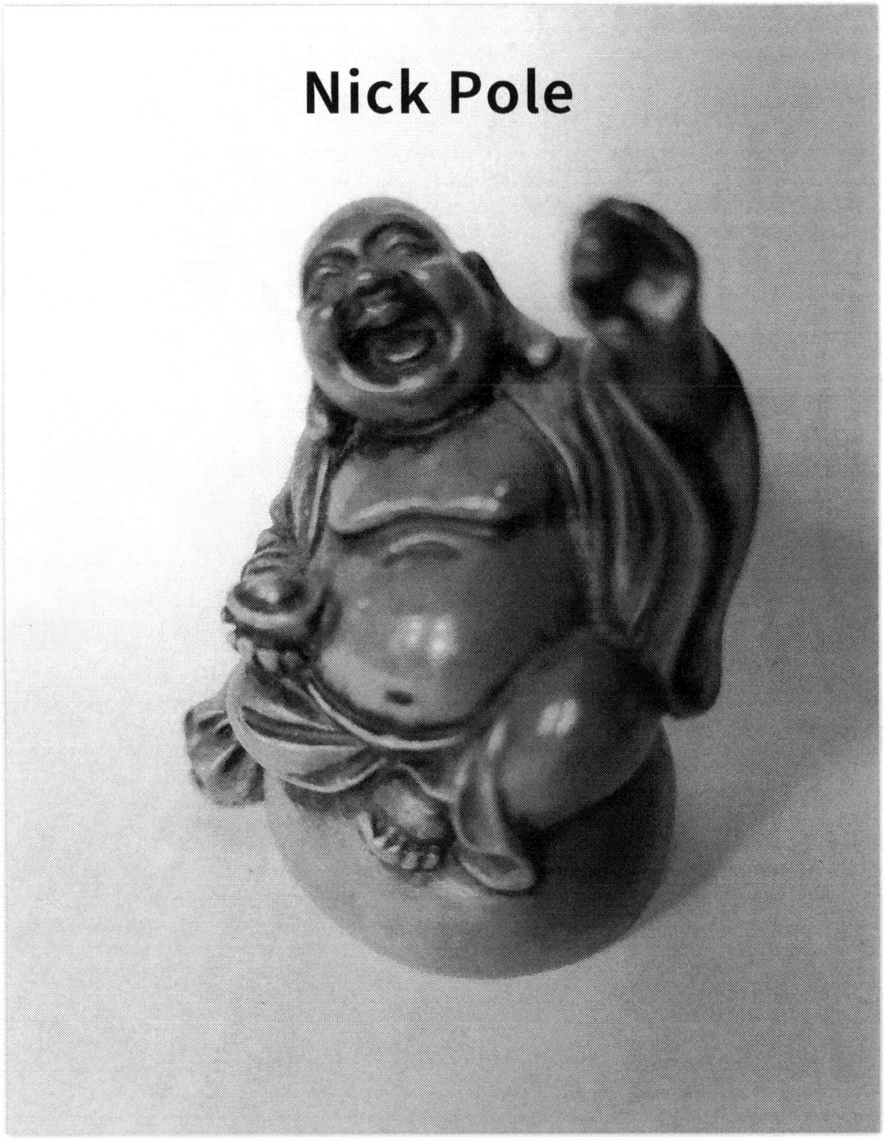

Zen, Shiatsu and the Art of the Clown

”From the Clown’s point of view, Non-Doing means never trying to solve a problem, but simply being with it, playing with it creatively until it finds some way to resolve itself. For me this is a perfect reminder of how we work in shiatsu, not pathologizing or trying to control the Qi, but simply being respectfully present with the energy in a system, and letting it make its own connections. That’s non-doing in action.

A Zen master is walking along the road. A Clown is coming in the other direction. They meet. How do they know which is the Zen master and which is the Clown? This is a koan I just came up with, inspired by the extraordinary life of Bernie Glassman, whose combination of Zen and clowning suggests some fascinating possibilities for how we might think about shiatsu. From a New York Jewish background, Glassman found himself drawn to the study of Zen in the 1970s when interest in it was just beginning its exponential growth in American popular consciousness. Working in Los Angeles as an aeronautics engineer, he became a student of Maezumi Roshi, an intense young Japanese Zen priest who had learned English as a boy by hanging out with the occupying American soldiers billeted at his father's Zen temple in Japan. Glassman plunged into Zen, studying with Maezumi for fifteen years and becoming ordained as a Zen priest himself. Soon after that he got into trouble with many in the Zen establishment by pursuing his own more socially-engaged form of Buddhism. Returning to New York, he set up a bakery to help unemployed people back into work, which eventually turned into a multi-million dollar philanthropic enterprise. Later, he co-founded Zen Peacemakers, an international group dedicated to bringing witnessing and healing to sites of conflict and suffering, including annual visits to Auschwitz with multi-faith groups.

From Trauma to Clowning

So how did he become a Clown? In interviews, he says it was when he noticed that the people he appointed to responsible positions in Zen organizations were taking themselves too seriously. He needed some way to help them lighten up. That no doubt is one reason and it points to one of the key principles of clowning – and shiatsu – never try to solve problems, just play with them until they solve themselves. But a glance at Glassman's biography shows that there was almost certainly more to it than that. In the space of just three years before he took up clowning, he suffered two traumatic bereavements. In 1995 his teacher Maezumi died suddenly and bafflingly – almost certainly a suicide – leaving a will that appointed Glassman as the head of his White Plumb community. Then in 1998, after Glassman had just moved from New York to New Mexico with his wife, the Zen teacher Sandra Jishu Holmes, to a house she had set her heart on as a peaceful and beautiful sanctuary from the demands of their twin careers, she had a heart attack and died, aged only 57. Shocked to the core, Glassman – whose diary was usually fully booked two years ahead, cancelled all his commitments and simply sat with his grief for as long as it took.

Soon after that, his study of clowning began. The teacher he found was Moshe Cohen, who had not only studied classical and modern European clowning, but also Japanese Kyōgen, a kind of comic antidote to the formality of Nōh theatre, and Butoh, the modern Japanese dance form noted for its utter physicality and raw emotional honesty. Perhaps it was his commitment to that same sort of honesty that drew Glassman to clowning, where whatever happens on stage, you accept it, welcome it, play with it, build on it. This clearly resonated with Glassman, the socially engaged Buddhist and peace activist. The trips he organized to Auschwitz with groups that included the children of both camp survivors and SS guards who had worked there, were about finding ways as a group together to witness and accept everything that had happened, to find a common humanity and a compassionate connection in the face of the worst that humanity can do.

For his part, Cohen found having a Zen master for a student transformed his teaching. Up till then he had concentrated on training performing artists. Within a couple of years, he and Glassman began teaching Clowning Your Zen workshops, helping everyone from Buddhist monks to corporate teams if not to become enlightened then at least to ›lighten up‹, to use the basic principles of clowning to develop more mindful and collaborative ways of communicating with each other, caring for each other and looking after themselves.

The Zen Clown Does Shiatsu

So what would happen if we bring this Zen Clown approach to the way we learn, teach and practice shiatsu? Let's look at four basic principles and how we might apply them. The first we could call Emptiness. In the purest form of clowning, you come onto the stage with no script, no agenda, no plan and no ego. You are simply there, present, listening with your whole body, ready to respond. The space you enter is also empty, except for some simple object – a piece of cloth on the floor, a chair, a broom. Your task is simply to engage authentically with whatever you find there. Peter Brook, one of the most innovative theatre directors of his generation, begins his book *The Empty Space* by saying that any empty space becomes a stage as soon as someone walks across it while someone else is watching. In shiatsu, as soon as a client enters the empty space which I am holding for them, something begins to happen. That something may be subtle and may be easily missed, which is why the clown – like the shiatsu practitioner – needs to listen with the whole body. The more embodied we are, as Reg Ray says, in *Touching Enlightenment*: »The more we uncover a vast and expanding interpersonal world of connection with other people… the more we sense others as inseparable from ourself.« And the Buddhist scholar Stephen Batchelor has pointed out that this kind of embodied awareness is what the Buddha himself originally meant when he said: »I mainly dwell by dwelling in emptiness … «, not a negation of self but fully inhabiting the embodied space of one's sensory experience, undisturbed by habitual reactions. »To dwell in emptiness«, Batchelor says, »brings us firmly down to earth and back to our bodies. It is a way of enabling us to open our eyes and see ordinary things as though for the first time.« That is definitely the kind of emptiness the Zen clown aims to dwell in.

»Yes, and …«

We could call the second skill ›Acceptance‹. But in clowning that slightly bland, do-goody noun transforms into the energetic affirmative ›Yes, and …‹. The core interactive skill in clowning, as in every form of theatrical improvisation, is the ability to say ›Yes‹ to whatever your clowning partner, (or in our case, the shiatsu client) offers. Clowns feel all emotions, more deeply than anyone else, but they also have the skill to stay with those emotions without suppressing or ignoring them, until something positive can surface from the depths. ›Yes, and …‹ is an extraordinarily powerful way to amplify conversational connection, or in the case of shiatsu, your connection with Qi. If I remember ›Yes, and …‹ as I touch my client, it reminds me to be not just open but appreciative, in an almost aesthetic way, to what my senses are telling me about this point and this person, and it empowers the client's Qi to communicate back to me in the most direct and honest way. In effect, ›Yes, and …‹ is a mindfulness practice in itself.

The third space, ›Not Knowing‹, is a continuation of that meditative connection. Allowing yourself not to know any of the things that you think you ought to know is like swimming underwater, suspended in a completely different element, where none of the sounds from the surface world can distract you and you are free to focus completely on your direct sensory experience. In both clowning and shiatsu it's a reminder that knowing doesn't come from the head and that it's time to come back to whole body listening; an invitation to open ourselves to pure ›Beginner's Mind‹ where there are no maps or preconceived notions whatsoever. Of course in clinical shiatsu we need our expert mind, with its left-brain ability to give things names and to put them into categories. Language allows us to conceptualize, to manipulate and edit our experience, to make the kind of connections that we couldn't make if we lived, as mindfulness sometimes seems to imply we should, entirely ›in the moment‹. But language also separates us from our direct experience of the thing that is named and in shiatsu we need that more than anything else. Touch brings us back to the bodymind and to the right brain's capacity for empathic connection. Stephen Batchelor describes this as: »A vivid alertness that … hovers on the cusp between ›it is‹ and ›it is not‹, resisting the seductive lure of certainty.« This space of Not Knowing, then, is an invitation to train ourselves to be able to inhabit, or be inhabited by, the emptiness that is there before any names or labels come, (always remembering of course that ›emptiness‹ is also just another name).

Playing, not Fixing

The fourth principle, ›Non-Doing‹, may seem a paradoxical way to describe the playfulness that is the trademark of the clown, but it is also the core message of the Dao De Jing, the original textbook about how Qi works, which though it is not often described as such, is a very playful book. Who but a clown would start by telling you that the subject of their book is impossible to write about? From the Clown's point of view, Non-Doing means never trying to solve a problem, but simply being with it, playing with it creatively until it finds some way to resolve itself. For me this is a perfect reminder of how we work in shiatsu, not pathologizing or trying to control the Qi, but simply being respectfully present with the energy in a system, and letting it make its own connections. That's non-doing in action.

In his late seventies, Glassman had a stroke that severely affected the right side of his body and his speech. Applying his Zen Clown principles to what life had just thrown at him, he worked every day with Feldenkrais exercises, which include frequent periods of rest to allow the brain to process what the body has just done. In these rest times Glassman found himself in a profound state of Not Knowing, at a level he had never experienced before. He surprised his rehab therapists at the pace at which he was able to recover both movement and speech. Back home months later, some friends came to visit and in the conversation someone asked him, as someone usually does in these stories, »What is the essence of Zen?« Glassman looked at her and realized that, even though he had fully recovered his speech, he had no idea what to say. He had been asked the question countless times and never had any trouble answering it; now all he knew was that he could feel it, but had no words to describe it. »What that did to me was huge«, he said later. »A huge sense of joy. Or a sense of holy cow! I don't know what this is, and now I can find out … that's what I remember, this state where I was just, wow. I have a new chance to clarify what does that mean.«

»One Continuous Mistake …«

In shiatsu, the verbal mind is always pulling us back into its own kind of thinking, into routine and technique, seeking certainty and wanting results. Zen originated as a reaction against this kind of thinking, and just as Zen has through the centuries found it necessary to refresh itself, (coming to the west was one way it did that), in shiatsu we can use the Zen Clown's principles to refresh our way of being with the client, coming back again and again to emptiness, saying ›Yes, and …‹ to whatever comes without needing to know what it is or how to describe it in words. And when it comes to playing creatively, there is one more secret ingredient: get yourself into trouble and be fearless about making mistakes. That's what makes clowns funny and, as the 13thC Zen master Dogen put it, »Zen is one continuous mistake«.

Literature

Brook Peter (2010): *Der leere Raum*. Alexander Verlag.

Ray, Reginald (2008): *Touching Enlightenment: Finding Realization in the Body.* Sounds True Inc.

9

Bill Palmer

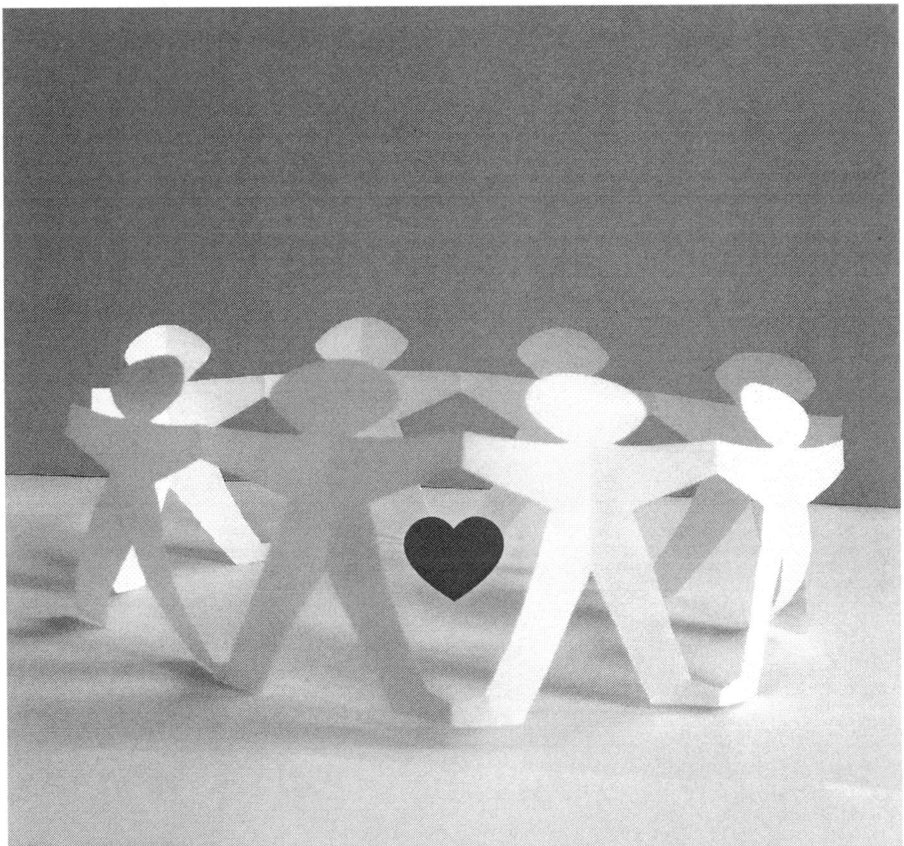

Muscles have Feelings too

" The key idea is to see each part of the person as a valuable part of a team, including the ›disabilities‹. The emphasis of the therapy then becomes to help the team to operate well together, rather than to change the individuals in the group.

The paradox of change

People come to therapy to change something. Maybe they want to get rid of pain or deal with emotional issues or cure an illness. They often feel powerless to deal with their condition themselves. Maybe they want the therapist to rescue them and make it go away but, even if they don't expect so much, the therapy is usually seen as a way of solving their problem.

This article explains why trying to change often doesn't work, particularly in long term, chronic situations. Paradoxically, letting go of the desire to be different can create a better environment for real improvement to happen spontaneously. I will also discuss how this change of focus could be good for the health of society.

For thirty years I have worked with »severely disabled« children. I find that many children with »disabilities« are traumatised by the orthodox therapy they receive because both the parents and the therapists feel a pressure to try to make the child develop as normally as possible. The fact that they are focusing on how to change the condition means that the child feels there is something wrong with her core self. The result is that she sees her disability as unacceptable and does not include in her view of herself the parts of her body that do not work *normally*. In my experience this often leads to the child growing up into a frustrated adult, feeling a helpless victim to their condition.

In contrast, when parents and therapists start to see a child as »whole« rather than disabled she relaxes into herself and from this ground she starts to explore how to develop her unique potential without comparing herself to the norm. The father of one of the children I work with recently wrote this poem to her:

when i am with you,
i am,
your hands and your voice,
i try to see how your every movement is a word,
how the sounds you make express the truth of your soul's feeling
your eyes show your sadness
and your joy
your smile radiates your blessing
on all of we
who do not understand
...

my prayer is not for your healing
for you are whole
my prayer is that i may grow to be strong enough
to hold the beauty of all you express
and help give it form

Rohan White, 2014

This viewpoint applies to everyone. People with a chronic condition frequently view it as a disability and, if it doesn't change, feel ashamed, disempowered and stressed. Much of the suffering associated with chronic issues comes from the frustrated desire to change rather than the condition itself. So how do we help a client to embrace themselves as they are without collapsing into a fatalistic acceptance of a situation that they feel powerless to change?

The individual as a team

The key idea is to see each part of the person as a valuable part of a team, including the »disabilities«. The emphasis of the therapy then becomes to help the team to operate well together, rather than to change the individuals in the group.

The idea that the self is a group has a long respected history in psychology (Carter) and transpersonal psychotherapy introduced the term »sub-personalities« to capture this idea. As Roberto Assagioli, originator of psychosynthesis, said: »We are not unified; we often feel that we are, because we do not have many bodies and many limbs, and because one hand doesn't usually hit the other. But, metaphorically, that is exactly what does happen within us. Several sub-personalities are continually scuffling: impulses, desires, principles, aspirations are engaged in an unceasing struggle.« (Kentaur Traening)

Therapies such as Voice Dialogue modify this idea of »unceasing struggle« by viewing the multiple selves as a community who can learn to communicate maturely and live together as equals. The advantage of seeing the personality as a community is that it gets to grips with the inevitable conflicts and differences within the self rather than aiming for a false harmony.

On the other hand, the philosophy underlying most body-therapies and physical medicine is that the body is a single organism whose constituent parts are mindless. From this viewpoint, there is no understanding of why a part of the body should resist harmonising with the whole. Physical therapists recognise that to re-pattern a habit may take some hard work but the basic viewpoint is that the parts of the body are naturally in harmony and need to be reminded, persuaded, manipulated and taught how to find this ideal state. There is often an implicit assumption that the body should be the servant of the mind and if it doesn't do what the mind wants then this is a problem.

Multiple minds, multiple bodies

But if the mind is multiple, there is no one ruler for the body to obey. Furthermore, the different sub-personalities sense themselves through the posture they assume and the way in which they move the body. So the many personalities are embodied in muscles, organs and fascia and the struggle between the personalities is reflected in conflicts within our anatomy. Because of this, I find it helpful to view the body as a community of autonomous agents rather than a unified machine and, since meridians are the connectors and communicators between different parts of the body, one can view Shiatsu as a pre-eminent »group therapy for the body«.

I imagine each part of the body as having personality and feelings of its own, not just being part of the embodiment of a sub-personality. A chronically tense muscle may be *sulky* and resist relaxation until its feelings have been understood. Instead of trying to relax the muscle, it may be important to acknowledge its tension and respect its grievance. In touching such a muscle I imagine I am listening to a friend with a valid complaint. This viewpoint changes the quality of touch and helps that part of the body to feel heard and seen as a valuable member of the group.

This is the basic philosophy of Movement Shiatsu: to see the body as a community and to help this community to live together with respect and awareness. In practice, there are two complementary approaches to helping this body-community to live together that I call »Including the Kyo« and »Assisting the Jitsu«.

Including the Kyo

The concepts of Kyo and Jitsu, which we normally use to describe the state of surface meridians, can be extended to apply to these body-group members. As I have explored in a previous article (Palmer, 2013), the Japanese character for Jitsu means »That which is shown« while the character for Kyo means »That which is hidden«. So although a Kyo meridian may be *empty* the Ki of the meridian is only hidden and its hiding place is usually a part of the body that is immobilised or not joining in with the activity of the rest of the community.

This uncooperative part can seem like an obstacle to the rest of the group and there is a tendency to reject it or drag it along. But this breaks the team spirit. It's like a group of people who are climbing a mountain. If one person is injured then that person puts a strain on the rest of the group. Maybe they have to carry them, and the injured person feels ashamed and stressed themselves for holding up the group. But this dynamic of stressed Kyo/Jitsu is only maintained if the group still has the aim of climbing the mountain. If, instead, they decide to change the game and change their aim to »having a picnic« then everyone can take part, the group is not stressed and the injured party has time to heal without feeling bad about sabotaging the group aim.

True healing takes place if the rest of the group pays attention to the Kyo part and changes the game in such a way that it can join in.

This is consistent with the Zen Shiatsu paradigm of helping the Ki of the Jitsu meridian to support the Kyo meridian. But in chronic situations, I find it is not enough to work only with meridians; the Kyo has become embodied in a *hidden* part of the body and is resistant to change because it doesn't feel included. To melt this resistance, the person needs to become aware of that part themselves and to change the way in which they use their body to include and care for it.

The desire to fix a disabled part that is not ready to get better can actually inhibit healing because that part feels bad about itself and becomes more deeply hidden. Because it hides itself, the rest of the group does not take care of it, so it remains under strain. Letting go of the desire to change creates an environment where the Kyo part can feel better about itself and come out of hiding to join in with the others.

Assisting the Jitsu

In real life, people often can't change the game to care for the Kyo. They have jobs to do, children to care for and relationships to maintain. They can't just stop all this to »have a picnic« to include it. But if we see the Kyo as a valuable part of the team who can't join the game at the moment and view the Jitsu as the substitute who has the energy to compensate for its inactivity, then the process of treatment is transformed.

In a football team, if the striker is taken off because of injury and someone, whose speciality is defence, is the only one available as a substitute then the replacement will be hard pressed to fill the role of the one taken off, and will feel under pressure and tense. However, if the whole team shares the job of filling the striker's role, then everything works smoothly and with good heart.

This metaphor exactly describes what can happen in the body. If a part of the body is vulnerable and needs to be taken off the pitch, then another part will try to take its place and may become stressed in the process. But if the rest of the Person-Team can help in the process of compensation then the stress disappears.

Movement Shiatsu has specific techniques for facilitating this by bringing awareness to the way in which the neighbouring parts of the body are communicating with the Jitsu area and helping the neighbours to move with it. This, in turn, highlights how more distant areas can assist the movement until the whole body is included in supporting the Jitsu. I view the traditional meridians as innate maps tracing chains of supportive connection between members of the body community; but we also create new pathways as we develop. I like to think that I am helping a client to create new meridians, not just working with the ones in the books.

Is this approach effective?

Psychological therapies such as Cognitive Behavioural Therapy (CBT), Neurolinguistic programming (NLP) and Emotional Freedom Techniques (EFT Tapping) explicitly concentrate on changing behaviours and have a good track record for treating people with debilitating phobias. Many body therapies also focus on change, adjustment and intervention with good success. So what is the point of the approach I have been advocating? Is it effective and when is it appropriate?

I think this is a fundamental question, which resonates with many of the issues facing modern society. Essentially, I feel that this approach is especially appropriate in situations in which the client has to live with and be creative with their condition rather than change it. For instance, old age, disability, degenerative conditions and other long term chronic issues.

Modern society is focused on consumption. Advertising makes us feel inadequate so that we will buy products that will change us. The whole media industry builds a picture of an ideal which most of us can't live up to. The result is that we are conditioned to see ourselves as needing change, and the quicker the better. So therapies that focus on change gain high status and conditions that are resistant to change are pushed under the carpet. The »broken« in society, including the insane, the elderly and the disabled are not seen as useful members and their potential value is ignored.

Blessed are the cracked for they let in the light!

But all of us are broken in some way. The personal growth movement focuses on positively mending these weaknesses and thus gaining »empowerment«, »healing« and »transformation«. So parts that remain disempowered and do not improve feel particularly bad about themselves because they don't take the opportunity that personal growth systems offer!

In my lifetime, I have seen society radically change. In the 1970's, most of my contemporaries were interested in the deep problems facing humanity. We were starting to see the thoughtlessness of the human race and its danger to the planet and feeling the humbled by this view. Nowadays most of western societies seem to be driven by philosophies of dynamic individualism and the arrogance encouraged by the successes of technology. People are valued by their wealth and success rather than their contribution to others.

Therapy has also changed response to this sea change in society, becoming driven by the aim of fixing problems rather than developing awareness and care. This is reflected in a more superficial approach to ourselves: we are more concerned to look good than to be good and this undermines our compassion for each other. If our society focuses on fixing the blemishes and looking good while hiding the real issues, then we will treat our environment and each other in the same way. I can only see disaster and destruction if we continue to go that way.

Shiatsu and its philosophy of caring for the Kyo could be an environmentally friendly and spiritually effective therapy. As long as we don't try to fix the Kyo, but help it to feel a valuable part of the whole then we are healing a deep malaise in this society. Jesus of Nazareth said: »Blessed are the meek for they will inherit the earth.« An interpretation of this beatitude is that people who include and befriend their own weaknesses will have compassion for others and for the planet. In particular, insane, elderly and disabled people could be cherished by society because they show us how to live with things instead of trying to change them. It's only when we lose the arrogance that says we can fix everything that we will learn to be part of the planet rather than just to exploit it.

Bibliography

Campbell, Joseph (1992): *This Business of the Gods.* Windrose Pubns, Canada.

Carter, Rita (2008): *Multiplicity.* Little. Brown Spark, 1. Auflage.

Ferrucci, Piero (1997): *Werde was du bist.* Rowohlt Taschenbuch, S. 57.

Palmer, Bill (2013): *The Tiger in the Grove.* In: Shiatsu Society Journal.

Hobbs, Jeremy (2013): *Oxfam seeks new deal' on inequality from world leaders.* BBC Staff.

Kristof, Nicholas (2014): *An Idiot's Guide to Inequality.* In: New York Times.

Slater, John (2013): *Annual income of richest 100 people enough to end global poverty four times over.* Oxfam Report.

White, Rohan: *Erin Fae.* Unpublished Poem 2014.

World Economic Forum. Global Risks 2014.

10

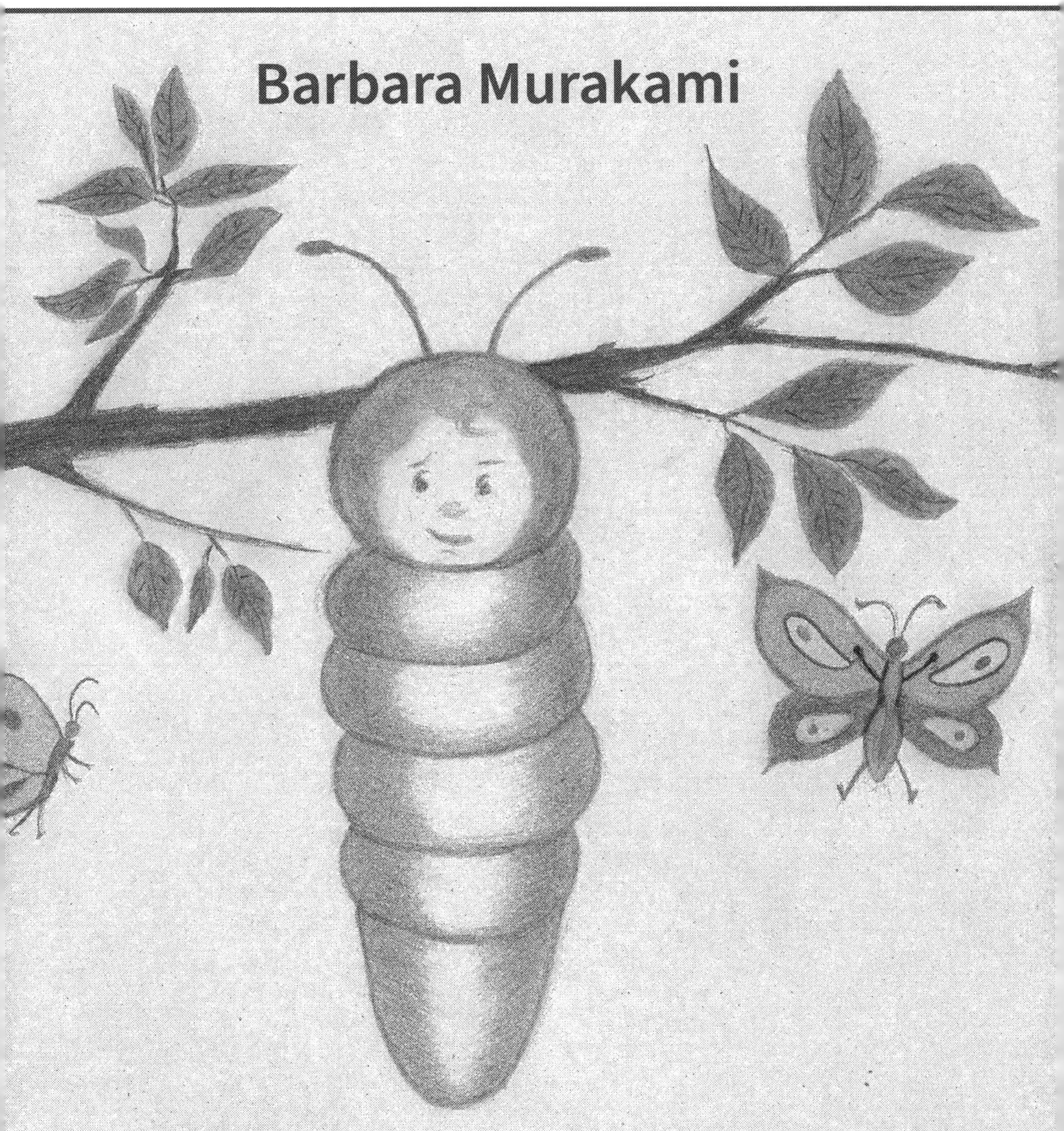

Like a Caterpillar in a Cocoon

Shiatsu for Children with Behavioural Problems

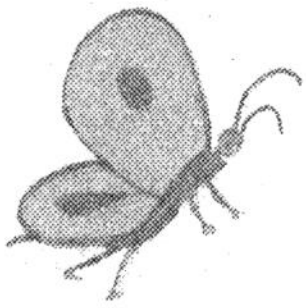

Children are Different

is the title of a book by the renowned educationalist Maria Montessori. Shiatsu sessions with children are also often very different from those with adults.

I wrote the text *Like a Caterpillar in a Cocoon* back in 2005 for the Journal of the German Shiatsu Society. The children in question are now adults. However, the essence of the text has lost none of its topicality. That is why I am happy to make it available for this book.

I have been working full-time as a teacher in a special school for educational support for 24 years. Shiatsu enables me to connect with children and adolescents on a level beyond the verbal. This is what I would like to talk about.

The Outer Framework

I am employed as a teacher at the Private Special School for Educational Support, run by the Graf-Recke-Foundation. The children who attend our school cannot be adequately supported in a regular school setting. They exhibit extreme behavioural challenges in social, emotional, psychosomatic and/or psychomotor areas. Their school performance is also often far from adequate. Many are highly aggressive, disoriented and uncontrolled, while others are anxious, passive and inhibited. The majority of the pupils live in a home associated with the school due to many different serious family problems. More and more children come directly from most difficult life circumstances (experience of abuse or maltreatment, extreme neglect, frequent changes of caregivers etc.). And more and more children have spent a shorter or longer period of time in psychiatric care before being admitted. They are between 6 and 13 years old.

In my role as a teacher, my primary task is of course to »teach the children something«, that is, to impart knowledge. This is no different at a special school. However, education is not just about knowledge that can be tested, it is also about social and emotional development, promoting perception and motor skills. And our pupils find it particularly difficult to engage with learning material at all. Too many obstacles stand in their way. This is where Shiatsu comes in. Therefore, I gradually created spaces and times in which Shiatsu could be integrated into our work.

- In our school, there is a concept for special educational needs lessons with individual pupils or with small groups of pupils. They usually take place at the end of the morning or in the afternoon.
- During the school morning, there are always periods when the pupils work independently on freely chosen or assigned tasks. During these periods, there is sometimes an opportunity for short Shiatsu treatments.

- From time to time, I show the children simple Shiatsu techniques so that four or six of them can have ›treatments‹ simultaneously: I treat one of the boys, and another pair or two watch what I do and treat in parallel.

Most treatments take place on yoga mats in a corner of the classroom. For treatments outside school hours, I can use a room of the child psychotherapist who is employed in the home. ›Outsourcing‹ from the school building has advantages. It prevents role diffusion, and it minimises the reservations many children have towards anything associated with school.

A Little Practice

Kevin

Kevin is 11 years old. He lives in a residential group for hyperactive boys. He is the epitome of a fidgeter. In many situations he babbles on and on and can hardly sit on a chair for more than 5 minutes. Kevin isn't in my class. He comes to see me once a week for 45 minutes after school.

During his first visit, he naturally doesn't know what Shiatsu is, but he is very open and curious. I explain to him that there is an energy, similar to electricity, that flows through the body and keeps us moving. »In some places there is too much of it, then you are stiff or hyper, in other places there is too little, then you are limp.« I also explain to him that this energy flows through pathways that can be imagined as roads. »And sometimes, the roads are blocked or there are stones and rubble lying around. Then they have to be cleared so that the cars can drive again. Sometimes a road has potholes. Then you have to repair it. It is much the same with people. When the energy can't flow properly, you don't feel well.«

I ask Kevin if he would like to feel this energy. I guide him through an exercise that Akinobu Kishi called »Gyoki«: Kevin closes his eyes and gently places his palms together with a gap between them. He slowly increases and decreases the distance between his hands, trying to feel what is happening between them. »It's like a magnet!« he says in amazement.

Kevin complains of stomach pains. Because of the tablets (psychotropic drugs) he is given, his stomach sometimes closes up. However, he still feels hungry, hence the stomach pains.

Kevin lies down on his back. I hold the lower hara and lower back with both hands like a sandwich for a while and ask Kevin to say »now« when he feels the energy flow between my hands. This helps him with concentration and perception, and he enjoys it.

I run the ball of my hand several times with varying degrees of pressure over the stomach meridian on his leg, which feels full and hot. »Why don't you clean the road thoroughly in one place, but keep coming back?« Kevin wants to know. »I clean roughly first, then with a fine broom, then with a brush«, is my explanation, and Kevin is satisfied. During the foot rotation (we call it »roundabout«), Kevin first helps a lot before he can relax his foot.

Kevin asks many questions and talks loudly during the treatment of the front side. I turn him onto his stomach and he calms down. The treatment of the bladder meridian calms him even more and he doesn't say anything for a while. He particularly enjoys the ›Centipede‹ exercise: I take one foot in both hands, put the thumbs on the back of the foot, and let the fingers walk over the soles of the feet with some pressure.

In the supine position, I stroke his neck and let it rest quietly in my hands. Finally, I hold the »Third Eye« (the »off button for excitement«) for a while.

»How do you manage to get so calm?« Kevin asks with interest during our little conversation after the treatment. »I practise sitting quietly from time to time. Also, I receive Shiatsu treatments myself.« He then wants to know how much a Shiatsu treatment costs and is relieved to find out that he doesn't have to pay anything. »That gives me an advantage!«

As we say goodbye, Kevin clearly states that he enjoyed the treatment and would like to come back. »I can see that you really enjoy doing this. Really.«

5th Treatment

In the meantime, I had agreed with Kevin that he would draw a little picture of how he was feeling before and after each treatment. I always encourage children to do this. The pictures sometimes provide me with additional diagnostic clues. They give the children another way to express themselves and help them to improve their self-awareness and concentration.

Kevin draws a smiling stick figure. It has a big yellow dot on its tummy. The yellow dot is surrounded by small red dots. On the left there is also a green dot drawn. Kevin's comment: »Outwardly, I have a friendly face. Inside there is a lot of homesickness (the yellow dot). This is surrounded by a longing for home (the red dots). Green is joy, which I also have, but not as much.«

I ask Kevin where the homesickness is. He points to his stomach and heart area. »Like a block of ice«, he says. I suggest that maybe we could melt this block of ice. During the treatment (mainly on the stomach meridian) I stay with the image and tell a little story about it.

»If we want to melt the block of ice, we have to make a fire. First need thick branches (working on the thighs), then thinner branches (working on the shins) and small twigs (grabbing the toes). Now let's light the fire (rubbing the soles of the feet) and get it going with a bellows (both soles of my feet against my stomach). I think we need more wood (working on the other leg).«

»Now let's make the fire rise up to your belly (rubbing the legs, rubbing the stomach, resting the hands on the stomach). Now let's see if the ice melts and maybe gets so hot that it evaporates. You can then breathe out the steam with full power.«

Kevin clearly enjoys the treatment: »It's so cosy, I always like Shiatsu. It makes me feel so calm.«

Finally, he draws another smiling stick figure. The belly is all pink. The hands look like little suns with lots of rays. »Pink means all the feelings from before together, only in smaller amounts. And the hands are glowing hot.«

Said

Said is twelve years old. He has been known as the school bully for years. Just three months ago, he kicked a classmate who was already on the ground and gave the PE teacher who intervened such violent kicks that he had trouble getting out of the car for weeks.

The following short report is an example of small Shiatsu interventions in everyday school life.

There are twelve children in the room, each busy in their own way: two are playing checkers, two are watching them, one is reading, one is practising writing, two are doing maths, some are playing or learning on the computer. I sit at my desk writing in the class register. Said stands behind me and asks: »Can you give me a massage?« I let him lie down on a mat and massage his neck. After a while, he relaxes and I move on to the bladder meridian on his back. Finally, with a wink, I suggest: »I could show you something else you can do with your feet besides kicking.« I gently treat his feet and hands with the balls of my feet. Said looks very reverent. »May I try that on you?« So, I lie down on the mat and receive a very attentive neck, hand and foot treatment. After the lesson, Said comes past me briefly and gives me a hug.

Thomas

Thomas is also an eleven-year-old boy with hyperactive behaviour. Unlike Kevin, however, he is usually calmer from the outset during treatments. One of the most striking things about Thomas' behaviour is that he constantly and loudly expresses the feeling that he is not getting enough. If someone has ten potato crisps but he only has nine, there is a big commotion. If I praise another child, he immediately says: »And you don't say anything to me again.« And so on. He constantly feels hungry and is correspondingly overweight.

Thomas also drew a picture before and after each treatment. Before the first treatment, he uses a rainbow pen to draw a stick figure with a speech bubble: »I'm fine.«

Thomas spontaneously lies down on his stomach. I touch his back in two places. »It feels like you are touching my feet.« »Would you like that?« »Yes, very much.« So I treat his feet extensively, especially the kidney points. »I feel like a caterpillar crawling into a cocoon«, he murmurs. Shortly afterwards he falls asleep. He doesn't notice much from the treatment of the bladder meridian. When I turn him onto his back, he wakes up briefly but goes back to sleep right away. The stomach meridian feels very empty on his thigh and fuller on his lower leg. During the treatment of the stomach meridian and the Hara, his body moves involuntarily all the time. Thomas is surprised that the treatment is already over and wants more, how could it be otherwise? We agree that he can come back the following week. The stick figure Thomas draws at the end grins from ear to ear and says: »I'm more than fine.«

Thomas continued to fall asleep again and again during the following treatments. My attention was repeatedly on the stomach meridian, and it became possible to make Thomas more aware of his stomach-related issues such as wanting to have more and more. I soon showed him stretches for the stomach meridian. He obviously practised these at home too, because he proudly showed me his progress before each treatment.

The importance of Shiatsu in this context

Perhaps the previous practice reports have already illustrated what Shiatsu with these children can be about, apart from the specific meridian functions:

- The children I work with have often not experienced enough of the touch that is so crucially important for their emotional development or have experienced it in forms of violence and/or sexual abuse. The attentive, clear touch of Shiatsu can perhaps provide some compensation.

- Many of these children have not received and still do not receive enough attention from their caregivers. The mere fact that an adult gives them their undivided attention for half an hour or more is a surprising and joyful experience for them.

- Children with behavioural problems, especially hyperactive children, get into trouble everywhere and are often not welcome. The closeness that arises in a Shiatsu treatment can make them feel accepted for a while.

- I see deep-seated insecurity, a primal mistrust as a possible cause of hyperactivity.

- The deep pressure and the two-handed approach of Shiatsu can give children a sense of security and healing.

- In both adults and children, Shiatsu affects the limbic system, the area of the brain that regulates the endocrine, vegetative and psychic systems. It is the seat of emotions and controls emotional behaviour. Ryokyu Endo writes in his book *Tao Shiatsu*:

  »The limbic system is the repository of all the memories and special skills acquired through external experiences and childhood. This is why the limbic system is called the seat of the unconscious self. Stress, fear and anxiety confuse the limbic system, suppress autonomic nervous functions and internal secretions and reduce immunity to disease. (…). The limbic system is directly influenced by touching the skin. Therefore the even, constant pressure of Shiatsu not only relaxes the client and increases responsiveness, but also eliminates disorders in this part of the brain. Nerve tension is reflected in muscle tension, but the relaxation of the skin over the whole body caused by Shiatsu brings about catharsis and relaxation in the subconscious. One effect of Shiatsu is to help the client gain insight into the subconscious causes of their suffering. Through meridian therapy, clients are encouraged to face their problems without the interference of words.«[1]

This may partly explain the deep relaxation that can be observed in Shiatsu.

- Time and again, I have observed improved self-awareness in the children on various levels.

- When the children treat each other, they practise being mindful with each other and learn about other, non-aggressive forms of touch and contact.

Tips for Practice

- To help children concentrate on the shiatsu treatment, I sometimes use a singing bowl. I strike it and the child should keep their eyes closed until they can no longer hear anything. Sometimes their eyes remain closed afterwards.

- Children usually prefer broad pressure with the whole palm to punctiform pressure. Often this is more reassuring.

- Treatments for children are usually shorter. Some children only allow very short sequences, which can gradually be extended over time.

- With some children, but not all, I include little stories or images into the treatment. This can achieve various goals:

  1. Some children then find it easier to get involved.

  2. Ideas and symbols, especially when developed together with the children can provide them with better access to the unconscious. The language of images is a very ancient one.

[1] Ryoko Endo: *Tao Shiatsu.* 2002, S. 26

3. Recent research has shown that images have an organising power on a neurophysiological level. Body chemistry can change in a flash through visualisation. So working with the imagination is also effective on a biological level. The placebo effect is an example of this.

4. Images can help children to remember and anchor experiences they have had on a physical level.

- Many children do not easily accept direct touch, especially those with experiences of violence or abuse. Such children can initially be treated with a hedgehog ball, small or large sandbags placed on their bodies or through a blanket. And it is usually best to start with the periphery, i.e. the hands and feet.

- What should be a matter of course for all clients is particularly important for children who have experienced violence or abuse. It must be absolutely certain that nothing happens that the child does not want. Duration, position and pressure must also be fully adapted to the child's needs and not to our own ideas about what is good for the child or what a good Shiatsu treatment should look like.

- Most children prefer the treatment to follow the same routine every time. This is often particularly important for anxious or mentally less agile children.

- Children usually need a lot of stability. They may need to be held more, supported with pillows or a blanket or even treated on a beanbag.

Training of Caregivers

»If you want to build a ship, don't drum up your men to gather wood, divide the work, and give orders. Instead, teach them to yearn for the vast, endless sea.«

Antoine de Saint-Exupéry

In my role as a teacher, I can only treat a few children. However, treatments outside of my teaching hours are not yet funded. And parents of children who do not live in care homes often cannot afford Shiatsu treatments. In order to enable as many children as possible to experience Shiatsu, I have increasingly transitioned in recent years to teaching the basics of Shiatsu to educators, teachers, parents and other people who spend time with children either professionally or privately. These are mainly single weekends, sometimes with later refresher courses. This year, for the first time, I am organising a "Basic Shiatsu Training Course" over ten weekends for people who work with mentally disabled children or adults. The aim of these courses is to make participants aware of the importance of mindful touch, to familiarise them with simple techniques and to provide them with their own experiences with Shiatsu.

To illustrate how much can be achieved with these simple means let me share the story of a kindergarten teacher, which touched me and motivated me to continue on this path. Brigitte works in a kindergarten for mentally disabled children. Last year, she attended a Shiatsu course with me on a weekend. The bladder meridian was one of the topics. A few months later, she told me about a three-and-a-half-year-old boy with autism. Toilet training was currently the focus for this boy. While he still wore nappies at home, he no longer did so in kindergarten. However, the boy steadfastly refused to go to the toilet at kindergarten and held it in for the entire kindergarten day (9 am - 3 pm!). The first time Brigitte treated his bladder meridian, he relaxed so much that he urgently needed to pee immediately after the treatment and voluntarily went to the toilet with Brigitte. For a while, going to the toilet was always associated with a Shiatsu treatment. Now he can go without Shiatsu and the problem is solved.

Shiatsu is now a regular part of the programme at this kindergarten. The children love it.

11

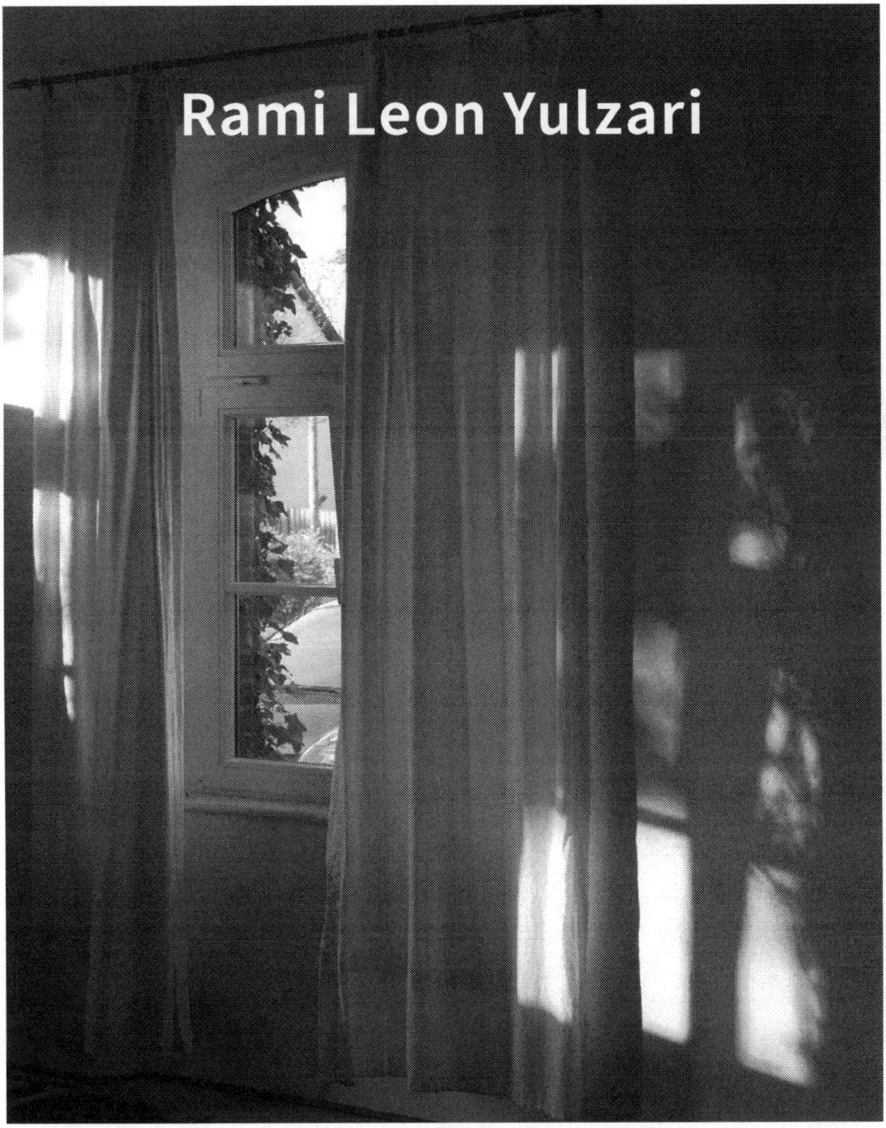

The Spirit of the Curtain
or
the Therapist contemplates

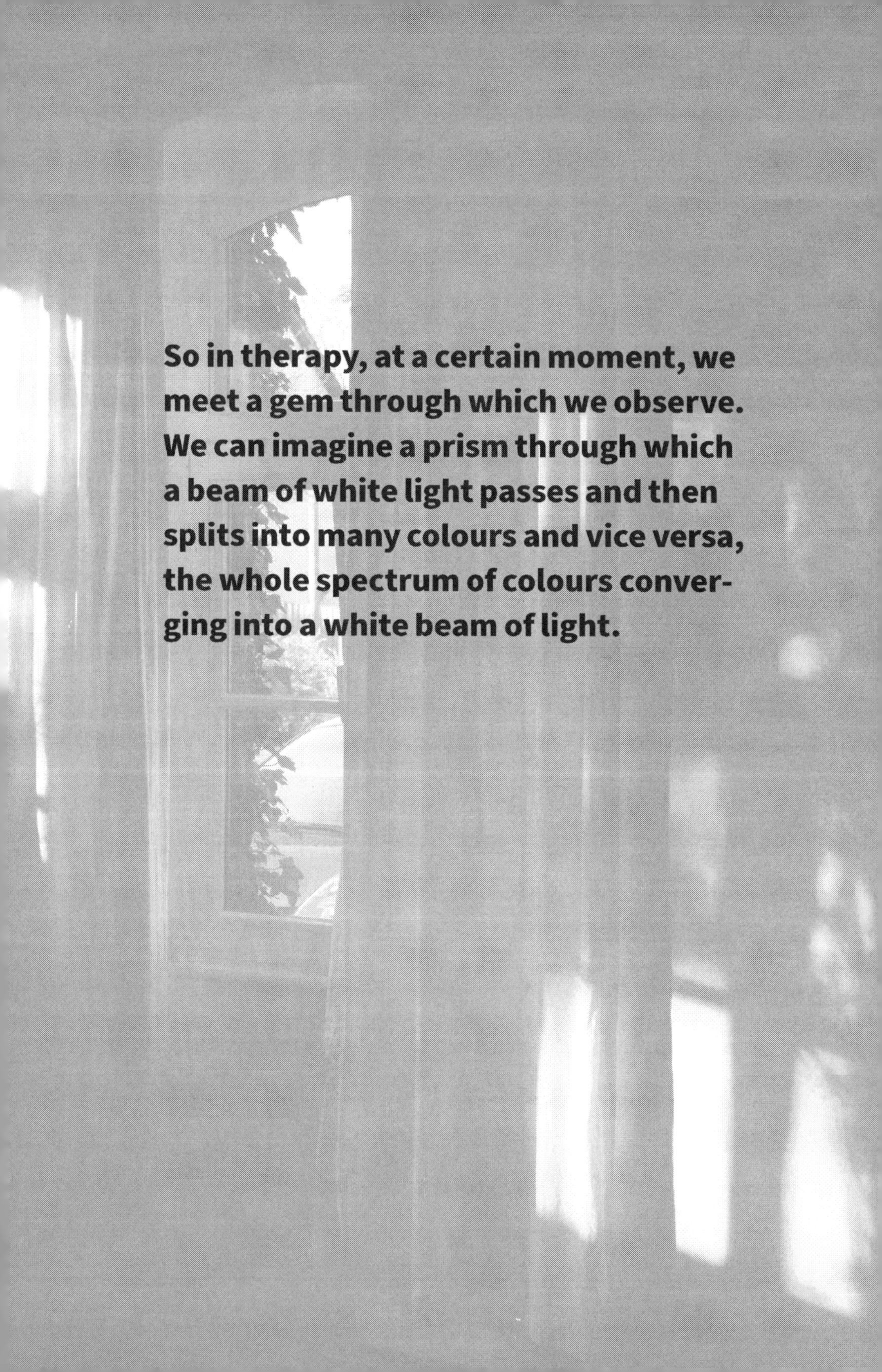

So in therapy, at a certain moment, we meet a gem through which we observe. We can imagine a prism through which a beam of white light passes and then splits into many colours and vice versa, the whole spectrum of colours converging into a white beam of light.

A plea

For someone to touch someone.

»The solution to the Zen riddle about the voice of a hand«, says Yoel Hoffman in his book *Moods*, »and also the solution to human suffering, which Sigmund Freud talked about, is that someone will touch someone and so on.« Someone who touches someone hears the sound that one hand makes when it claps and gets out of the circle of samsara, the circle of life and death, which is the circle of suffering. Like the Zen teacher Hakuin, who heard the cricket and all his doubts disappeared and his tears fell like waterfalls of pearls.

I also add: someone touches someone and hears the sound of the heart.

That someone touches someone seeps in, slowly, like a warm hand on a belly, creating ripples that, as they spread, change the heartbeat, cloud the thoughts and gather early morning dewdrops at the tip of the eye. And it enters at once, like the fox that creeps into the poet Ted Hughes in his poem *The Thought Fox*: »Till, with a sudden sharp hot stink of fox, it enters the dark hole of the head«.

That someone will touch someone.

When the secret is revealed, we discover that we have known it for some time, perhaps always. The answer seems to have been on the tip of our tongue all along and Yoel Hoffman takes it out of our mouths like a balloon coming out of a cartoon character's mouth and now it is real and it can be touched. I would add that someone will listen to someone and know where to touch and how to touch and the mystery will be solved. Then, whoever listens, will hear the sound of thunder on a clear day and the sound of emotions rising and falling and the sound of emotions swirling and spinning like a plastic bag in the wind and also those that pile up and gather dust. Those and those fall back to where they were, like a head that goes back to a socket in a pillow.

One might think, as the philosopher Charles Pierce did, that all things have a tendency to form habits, and a habit is the tendency to repeat a past action. Thus we can predict that a stone thrown from a height will fall to the ground, and also that the head will return to the pillow. We can predict sleeplessness, turning from side to side, the falling of thoughts from temple to temple, and the leaking of dreams onto the pillow. The puddles of dreams are the bed on which Zen riddles and dream interpretations grow, searching for meaning.

The therapist contemplates: People carry the circumstances of their lives like a chain around their necks until one of the vertebrae loosens or collapses. If we use the image of the rabbit hole into which Alice falls in Wonderland, we will find that those who fall into the hole grope around, looking for something to hold on to, collecting objects, emotions and feelings. Some of them have reasons, some are accidental, and all are temporary, but time, time sometimes turns and becomes a duration that can be called eternity. As in Alice Monroe's story *The Shining Houses*:

> »Here was no open or straightforward plan, no order that an outsider could understand; yet what was haphazard time had made final. The place had become fixed, impregnable, all its accumula-tions necessary, until it seemed that even the washtubs mops, couch springs and stacks of old police magazines on the back porch were there to stay.«

A plea rises through a window to heaven

In Chinese medicine, there is a group of acupuncture points whose quality is »window to heaven«. Their names include Heavenly Pillar, Heavenly Chimney, Door of Silence, Heavenly Pool and Spirit Palace. We can imagine a walk where we climb up the pillar, go up the chimney, open the Door of Silence, bathe in the Heavenly Pool and purify ourselves to come to the Palace of the Spirit. This is the way that connects earth and heaven, and if you think that there is separation, you can add body and soul. When we sail in our dreams, the »Window to Heaven« points will open a skylight through which our longing will rise to the place where longings are collected.

If we expand our consciousness through the window we can see the Diamond Sky in which Lucy lies; if we focus our consciousness and look closely we can see the matrix of the Diamond Sky which is Indra's web.

A Hindu myth says that the god Indra created the world by hanging infinite gems in heaven and they reflected each other infinitely in the infinite. This is the way our world is. Each time we meet a gem, it reflects all the others, and only from one angle. As human beings we can never see them all.

A human being is always finite, but at the same time its components are many, and in any case more than any other human being can ever see. When we meet the world, let us remember that we are looking at a gem that has many facets. When we meet a person, we want to remember that we are meeting a moment that contains great complexity.

The therapist contemplates: so in therapy, at a certain moment, we meet a gem through which we observe. We can imagine a prism through which a beam of white light passes and then splits into many colours and vice versa, the whole spectrum of colours converging into a white beam of light.

I remember a treatment, my hands resting on a patient and my eyes staring motionlessly at the curtain, seeing and not seeing. And more than seeing, they feel the movement of the curtain, a gentle, slow movement. The curtain is light, almost white, with tree branches with blurred edges, as if painted in watercolour on blotting paper, and they are silhouettes of a tree in the yard. The hem of the curtain is curled, touching and not touching the shadow of the curtain on the floor, and together, the curtain and its shadow move in perfect harmony.

How is the wonderful harmonious movement of the curtain and its shadow created? Could the patient and the therapist be so harmonious, even for a moment? How do we discover order and cyclicality in random movement? Do I see a curtain shadow as a curtain? Curtain as curtain shade? Or is it the spirit of the curtain or the Kami of the curtain? As in the Japanese Shinto religion, the Kami, the spirits of natural things, are the forces that control nature and explain the unexpected changes in it. In these moments of therapy, the curtain is present in our world, in the world of the patient and the therapist, like a mountain, like a tree, like a distant landscape, in which, if we look carefully, we can read meanings.

Is this a picture of the patient's life? Her eyes are closed and under her eyelids her pupils move in a random movement or a movement that, if we could speak its language, we could read her thoughts. Is this the history of the therapy? A map that is placed on the patient and guides the therapist along the path, which has latitudes and longitudes, names and reference points, each with a theory, that is, a name and characteristics and a course. On a winding road, perhaps up a mountain, where the weather changes, a wind blows, sometimes it comes from behind and pushes, sometimes it comes from the front and opposes. When it comes from the side, you sway more or less and have to stop to regain your balance, to hold your breath, to be in suspension before continuing.

The therapist contemplates: It is strange to be involved in things that are usually examined from the corner of the eye, through a glass, through a crack in the shutter. I look with open eyes at the movement of the patient‘s pupil. Her eyes are closed. She is neither asleep nor awake, an intimate half-sleep, usually hidden. Sometimes, inadvertently, it is exposed. Like when you hear the pianist Glenn Gould humming to himself as he plays Bach's Well-Tempered Clavier. Intimacy enters us without resistance and at once. A window to heaven is opened.
As in the poet Dalia Ravikovitch's poem *Alone with the poems*:

> »You sit in your room and the walls grow taller
> Colours deepen
> A blue kerchief becomes a deep well.«

If one were to lie on one's back with one's eyes on the ceiling, one would see indistinct forms forming there, whose movements are sometimes ordered and sometimes random, and which are airy and almost imperceptible to our senses. Like passing clouds, unreal, yet obscuring our vision, wetting our hands. Shadows on the ceiling become clouds. He says to himself: my back is on the bed, I lie in the room and there are its walls. What I see is a ceiling, and in the ceiling there are no clouds, and so he returns from his journey, landing on his senses. He is hungry or thirsty, he gets out of bed and goes to the kitchen. His wandering among the clouds remains like a slight headache, just above and between the eyes, where the mystics place the third eye, the one that sees beyond the horizon and even beyond the rainbow. It connects life stories to other worlds, where there is an explanation and a meaning for our lives, a language for our fears, for our pain and suffering, but also for joy, happiness and love.

A plea rises through a window to heaven and meets angels

The therapist contemplates (on the use of the word »strange«): Why strange? And what is strange? He recalls the psychoanalyst Jacques Lacan, in his twentieth seminar, called »More«, who said that strange (etrange) is like being an angel (etre-ange). Strange is like an angel looking down from the top of a cloud or the roof of a high building, seeing from afar, hearing from afar, not smelling, not touching.

Neither man nor God, has a father in heaven and no mother.

The singer Johnny Cash sang that there is no grave that can hold his body. When he hears the sound of the trumpet, »The trumpet, spreading a magical sound, among all the tombs of the world« (from the text of the Requiem, the Christian funeral service), calling all creation and all the dead to rise for the Day of Judgement, he will spread his wings and rise from the heavy earth. »Jesus«, he would say, »come and meet me in the middle of the air.« In the middle of the air, the meeting place of those who have wings and come from the earth and those who have wings and come from the sky. These are waving wings of water and these are waving wings of air, and so they connect air to water, singing songs of longing for the time before they were separated. When they separate, they are a pale shadow of themselves: the water moistens the sky and creates clouds that are reflected in the water, and when the clouds continue their journey, the water remains water.

The water receives moonlight, the shade of a tree, a rolling bridge, a bridge of barges and landing craft, even when they burn. Heavy smoke rises from them, then light smoke, then no smoke, and the water is still, a dragonfly flutters above it, a foot dips into it.

Water remains water, more stable and peaceful than the sun, more than delicate ships. As in W. H. Auden's poem *Musée de Beaux Arts*, which describes the fall of Icarus, the boy who wanted to be an angel, into the sea:

> »The sun shone
> As it had to on the white legs
> Disappearing into the green water;
> And the expensive delicate ship
> That must have seen
> Something amazing, a boy falling out of the sky,
> Had somewhere to get to and sailed calmly on.«

The expensive, delicate ship would be a rusty wreck in no time, suns collapse in on themselves and the water? Water remains water.
Zen master Dogen wrote:

> »The moon does not seek to be reflected in the water, nor does the water seek to reflect the moon.«

The fish swimming in the sea is not aware of the water, and the water in the sea is not aware of Icarus, his life and death. The water is in equanimity.

The therapist contemplates: Some practice equanimity to be water; some practice being water to be in equanimity. Some practice to be strong like a rock, and some practice to be strong like water. When you come to the treatment, be a rock that pours out water. When he leans over to drink the water, the patient might put an arm out and lean against the rock.

Plea descends from heaven on the wings of angels

Still, sometimes the rustle of life increases, humans are water only for the most part. When an angel falls into the water, there is excitement in the depths. He is received in the arms of soft seaweed, which place him on the soft, drowning sand until he disappears, leaving behind the imprint of his body.

The therapist contemplates: someone touches someone and finds traces of a body that has disappeared, signs of a past life. Smoke signals rise from invisible cracks. He listens to the whisper of coals.

Someone is touching someone, and the known becomes unknown, as in Alice Munro's story *Walker Brothers Cowboy*:

> »Like a landscape that has an enchantment on it, making it kindly, ordinary and familiar while you are looking at it, but once your back is turned, into something you will never know, with all kinds of weathers, and distances you cannot imagine.«

Someone touches someone else and remembers Shiki's haiku:

> »I look back –
> the man I just met
> has become mist«

Someone touches someone.

Light mist rises, mist that no one knows where it came from or where it is going, yet it surrounds the someone touches someone. As the eyes get used to it, shapes, images, visions and stories are revealed in the mist. What appears to be the end becomes the beginning and the possibility of change is revealed like the moon in the dark – it was always there, now it can be seen.

Bibliography

Hofmann, Yoel (2010): *Moods*. Keter Books, S. 95

Hughes, Ted (1996): *The Thought Fox*. Schoken Publishing House, S. 12-14

Munroe, Alice: *Tanz der seligen Geister*; Kindle Edition.

Ravikovich, Dahlia (1995): *You Must Remember. The Complete Poems Till Now.* Hakibbutz Hameuchad Publishing House, S. 115.

Shiki, Masaoka: *Selected Poems*. Columbia University Press, 1997.

12

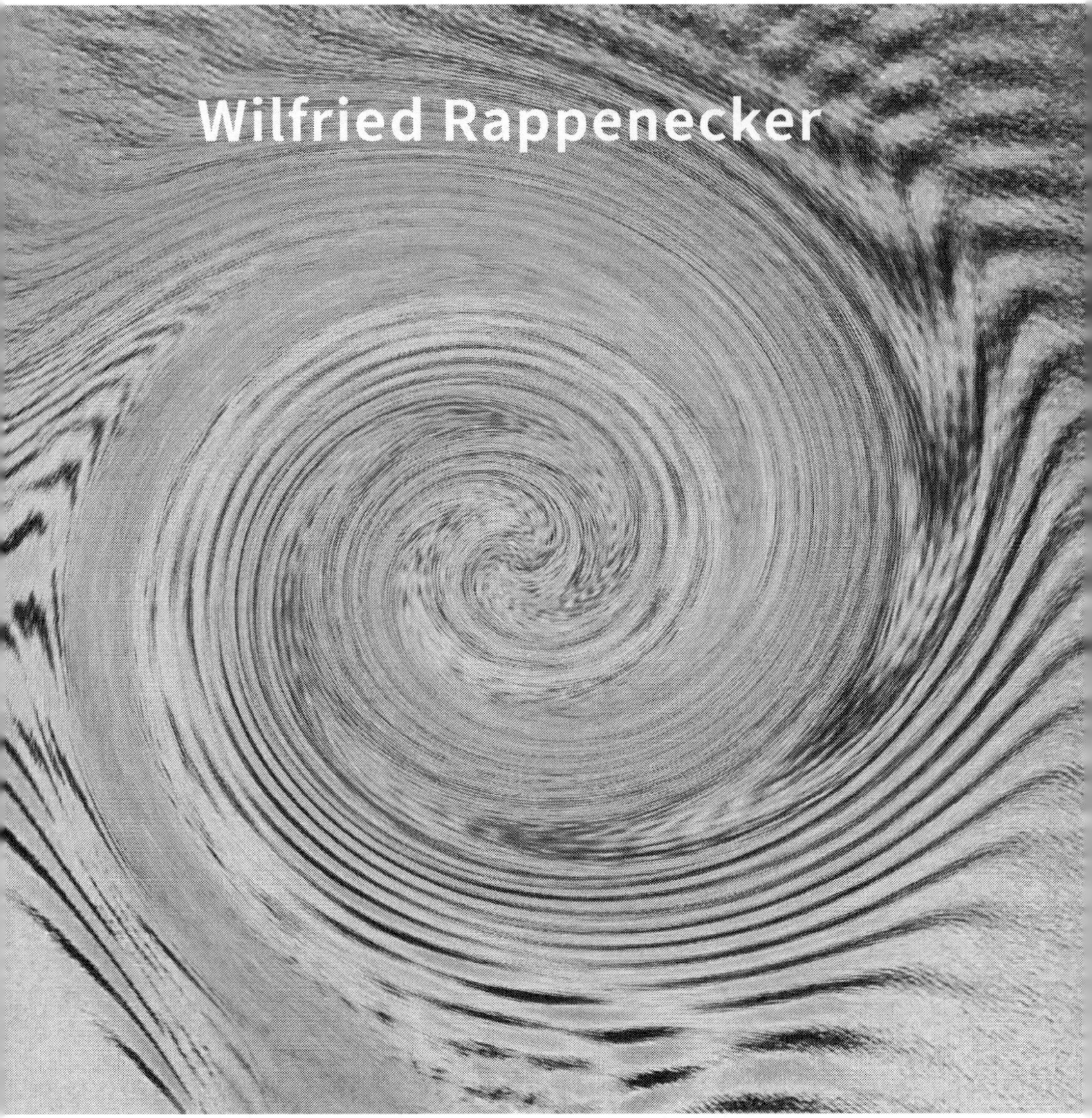

Resonance in Body Therapy

„ In bodywork, we describe resonance as a phenomenon that unfolds between therapist and patient. Mindfulness for oneself and being present in one's body on the part of the therapist is an important basis for resonance in a therapeutic setting.
Training and experience allow the therapist to amplify the resonance. However, the practitioner alone cannot generate resonance; the patient's response is essential. In this context, trust is an essential ingredient. The arising therapeutic space is more, and can facilitate more, than the space between two individuals who are not resonating with each other.
Resonance shapes, in one way or another, interpersonal communication. Resonance is the foundation for creating a sense of communion.

In Shiatsu, resonance describes a phenomenon which unfolds in every therapeutic situation between therapist and patient, and which is reflected in the therapist's perception of and the patient's reaction to the touch. Resonance always occurs when two people relate to each other. In this article I describe the effects of and prerequisites for amplified and deepened resonance as it occurs and can be promoted consciously in a Shiatsu treatment.

When resonance is amplified patients describe the effect of the touch as reaching significantly deeper, both physically and emotionally, than without deepened resonance. Clients relax more easily and deeply. The breathing becomes deeper, or lighter and shallower; there will be a perceptible decrease of both tissue and muscle tone; local tension dissolves.

In a state of amplified resonance, the therapist's perception expands from perceiving only the physical surface and superficially visible physical structures to perceiving the body-space, e.g. with a frozen shoulder, an injured knee or psychological complaints.

Being present in the body and the quality of attention

A state of increased resonance in this sense requires the practitioner »being present within himself«. This phrase describes a state in which the therapist perceives himself and his body in a relaxed way while being engaged in therapeutic interaction with the patient. This state is experienced as calm and centred – and felt as pleasant. The client, too, enters into a similar state, among other things through the deep relaxation experienced in the treatment.

Mindfulness towards oneself and being present in one's body is an indispensable basis for the therapist's mindfulness towards the patient and her body-space. This kind of mindfulness is not diffuse, but orientated and focussed. The fascinating combination of relaxed expansion and clear focus facilitates specific touch with nothing but focussed attention – together with manual touch; if considered appropriate, then also instead of it. This type of touch with attention is possible on any part of the body, on its surface as well as within the depth of the body-space.

It is interesting that even minor changes in the therapist's position, thinking or mental orientation can have a considerable influence on the resonance space formed together with the client. For example, if the practitioner straightens up and slightly expands himself during the touch, joints such as the shoulder joint and the wrist become permeable and the client will experience more freedom and lightness; and he will often become even more deeply relaxed. The client will experience the touch in different ways in his body, depending on whether the practitioner is working on an area with a well-defined focus of attention, or whether he is thinking of something completely different, such as his shopping list.

Expansive and focussed mindfulness can and must be learned and practiced. It is a kind of Qi Gong practice. Body exercises, such as Hatha Yoga and meditation, can play a decisive role in such training. The treatments themselves can be utilised as an effective practice for reaching a state of amplified resonance.

In the beginning it often requires courage to enter into a state where resonance is possible. It requires courage because it requires the practitioner to open up; to partially surrender the control of which aspect of myself emerges to the outside as well as the control of what can penetrate to the inside. To be in a state of resonance means that I show myself the way I am.

Therapeutic Space

However important it is that the therapist be able to enter into resonance – the practitioner alone can trigger the phenomenon we call resonance to only a limited extent. The client's response is essential. At that moment in the treatment, when the client relaxes, she opens herself up to the touch and establishes a connection with – and perceptible by – the therapist. This connection is a phenomenon of resonance, which people who are in tune with their bodies (e.g. bodyworkers, yoga practitioners, professional dancers or actors) will perceive much quicker and more strongly. This makes working with such people easier and more satisfying for the practitioner.

In the connection described here the feeling arises as if therapist and patient share a common space. At our institute we call this resonance space the Therapeutic Space. Training and experience on the part of the practitioner make it easier for this space to arise.

Trust is an essential ingredient of the resonance space described above. The practitioner's mindful touch and his relaxed presence allow the patient to relax and trust the setting and the touch. Trust increases the potential for resonance in the human system and thus its strength. Trust, therefore, facilitates an inner state in which words and touch have a deeper effect and support self-regulation and self-healing. In my view, this is an important component of any therapeutic effect (also in the context of a conventional medical intervention, as any G.P. in medicine knows) and one of the foundations of the placebo effect.

Not every client is able to open up to the emerging resonance space straight away. For example, offering this space to traumatised persons can trigger fear and a closing-up. In such cases, the therapist's experience is of great importance in order to continue offering openness and acceptance unilaterally, while at the same time understanding and respecting the client's closing up as a necessary act at that moment.

In the Therapeutic Space therapist and patient communicate with each other. Verbal and especially non-verbal information becomes accessible; information which goes beyond merely physical impressions and encompasses emotional aspects as well as aspects of the client's life history. Generally, based on his training and professional experience, the therapist can consciously use this information for working with the client. Due to the nature of resonance, clients equally receive information about the therapist but are usually unaware of this. Both transference and counter-transference are phenomena of the Therapeutic (Resonance) Space.

In a safe treatment setting the Therapeutic Resonance Space develops spontaneously and without any conscious action of the persons involved. However, it can also be induced by the practitioner based on her training and experience. Of importance are skilful perception, mindful approach and respect for the patient's integrity. Only then a therapeutic setting will develop that differs fundamentally from a non-resonating one.

Resonance in everyday life

What I refer to as the Therapeutic Space, in my view and experience, exists in every interpersonal communication. Language is only one of the essential tools for communication and together with gestures, facial expression and body language as well as the many ways of communicating, influences and shapes the communal space formed by human beings when they consciously or unconsciously relate to each other.

I presume that mutually experiencing and relating to each other in the Resonance Space also plays a great, if not central, role in people's everyday life; that it forms the basis for all important decisions; and that it brings the colour to our lives which we experience in our togetherness with others. Resonance is a foundation for a sense of communion.

Attempting an explanation

In attempting to find an explanation for the phenomena observed in bodywork as described above, the term »resonance«, borrowed from quantum/particle physics, appears very useful to me. Resonance arises when two vibratory bodies or spaces relate to and influence each other. In this concept, the human being as a whole (i.e. the human body, possibly including its surrounding space, as well as feelings and thoughts) is seen as a space capable of resonance.

In bodywork, a relaxed upright body, which »shows itself« and can openly enter into resonance, is therefore of great importance. Marked tension in the practitioner's body (e.g. in the shoulders, the neck or the wrists) will cause a constraint of the resonance space.

The less the vibrational capacity is impaired, the easier it will be for vibrational spaces to resonate with each other. Typical dampening factors in the human body are tension as a result of stress, anxiety, ambition etc. If the body suppresses certain painful experiences and if this suppression is permanently stored, there will be blockages on both an emotional and physical level. These can severely restrict the system's vibrational capacity. This applies to almost all people, but in particular to those with e.g. a neurotic or post-traumatic stress disorder or with borderline personalities.

Bodywork such as Shiatsu, but also psychotherapy, pursues the goal of dissolving such blockages and increasing the vibrational capacity of a person's entire system. If the vibrational capacity of a client's system increases during treatment, it is easier to find solutions to the current problem.

13

Rami Leon Yulzari

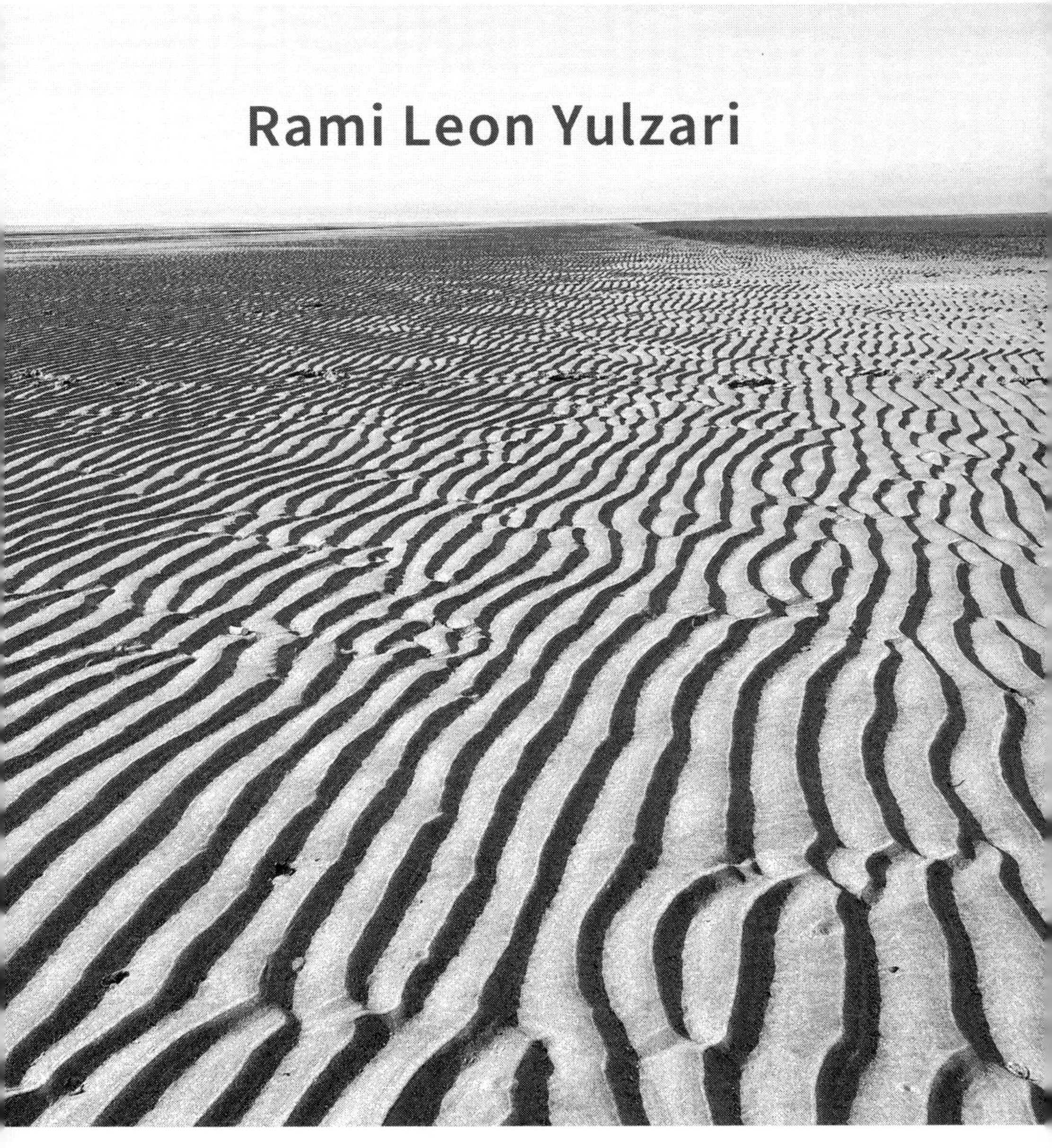

Images of Resonance

” I see Rembrandt looking at himself, the colour of his gaze is brown-black, the colour of the heavy earth into which he walks. When Rembrandt looks at me looking at him, his eyes are painted golden brown, the colour of compassion.

Photographs

Her nose looks as if it has collapsed to the side and her left nostril has shrunk into a crack. I watch closely as the air struggles to get in and out. There is fatigue in her breath. Through the window, against the grey sky, I see the deep green, almost black, of the top of the cypress swaying in the strong wind.

The cypress avenue leads to the riverbank where the ferryman waits. He takes those who come to him to the place where time ends. When he turns his head, I see his face and shudder. I am reminded of Sigmund Freud, who one night, in his sleeping compartment on a train, saw an old man in a nightcap and felt a great fear, which only increased when he realised that it was himself in the mirror.

It is winter now, I say to myself, and soon spring will come, the wind will die down and the cypress will return to its silent position. I feel my forehead widen and the tension in my jaw release. I accept that this is how she breathes. I trust her breath to take the air to its place.

The ferryman is waiting.

The sound of the clock is louder today. I wonder if the room is quieter today, or if the sound of the clock has increased. The throbbing artery at the side of her neck is more prominent today. Its beats rattle the fine wrinkles around it. I wonder if her heart is responding to the ticking of the clock. I wonder if the clock is ticking her heart.

Time, its mother Earth and its father Heaven, swallows the metronome, the echo of the church bells, the sliding snail, the delayed blossoming of the bougainvillea, the bare cherry tree, the cat whose nose is cold, whose sweat is cold, whose hind legs are paralyzed, the cat that whimpers weakly, whose eyes are frozen, and my hand on its belly was not enough, was not warm enough, was not big enough, was not wide enough, my hand on its belly was not enough, all are its children.

I can see, right in front of my eyes, the boy standing on the platform of the train, taking photographs. It was in the morning. In the evening they beat him to death. Imagine beating a little boy to death. It was such a time, you say, there are such times. The sun is shining and he is wearing a cap. There is no film in the camera, but he is enthusiastically taking pictures. He is happy. If he had not been beaten to death, he might have been taking pictures in the great parks of London, like the photographer who took pictures of a couple in love in the trees and found a body, or he might have been taking pictures in the gardens of Paris, watching the light at dusk melt into the fair hair of a girl and create a halo around her head.

Her arms are so thin, so light. They should be placed very carefully, first the elbow and then the hand, slowly. Her skin is white and almost translucent. The capillaries float beneath it like fish in an aquarium. It had been a long time since my mother had shown me a Japanese porcelain cup. If you hold it up against the light, the bottom of the cup becomes transparent and the face of a geisha appears. She told me to listen to the sound of a violin coming from a radio in a nearby room and her eyes moved away.

If a dead man‘s lips dropped in, what do they put in his mouth? If the last word, just before death, is „hands“, what was the first word? Who watches over the dead? and after death?

Sky above earth bellow, in the middle of the air find ground. Plant a tree, listen to children‘s voices as they play. Touch someone. Come back home.

Signs

It is the nerve, he said, pain comes from pressure on the nerve. It is sadness, I said, and I could see the tears pouring into his head and down his body and their water seeping through even the densest organs until they gather in the water basins where they dry and become lumps of salt of many sizes and shapes and shades, all pain.

I put your hand on mine. When your hand rests on my hand, the fingers that were clenched in a fist open up. The fingers have their own movement, like weeds in the wind. I see the marks of the nails that were notched into the skin, creating new stations on the paths of the palm.

He is lying on his back. He has thoughts of separation. If his eyes were open, he could see a map of his life with its main roads and side roads and paths and on all of them landmarks that are separations, screened on the curtain.

I look at the curtain. It has signs. If you know how to read them, you can see the line of life with the signs of separation and how the end appears at the beginning.

A light breeze blows through the weeds. As they move, a snake's slough is exposed, its skin wrinkled like the necks of people lying on the weeds, their faces in the ground, their backs to the sun.

The sand touched your body did you hold your breath there was no sign the skin did not move did not move the sand that touched your body are the organs joining are they separating yes they are separating are we going far?

So they parted: he said I love you, and at once the pigeons were released from their cages, and the hawks and the vultures, and the cries of the birds filled her head morning and evening and night, and her dreams were filled with the cries of babies she had not had.

His head is tilted back on the pillow and his mouth is wide open. He is breathing heavily. He looks like a drowning man who has managed to get his head out of the water. Then he is lying on the beach and water is coming out of his mouth.

One of my hands rests on the chest, moving with the movement of the breath. My other hand touches the root of the palm, paying attention to the pulse. As they pass through the centre of my chest, the rhythm of the breath and the pulse unite into one beat. I expand.

As time passes people come people go sometimes they leave marks bare rocks desolated cliffs places where only vultures live supreme creatures as vultures pass.

Glances

I look at her eyes in wonder, how they float in the skull cavities like lakes in a volcano. When thoughts of her dead son come to her, flames rise from the depths and the boiling lava flows into her eyes.

Her eyes will soon be ashes, and so will her lips, which converge into her mouth.

I cover her eyes with my hands. She sinks into the warm darkness. I slide the tips of my fingers over her eyelids, remembering the cat licking the inflamed eyes of a kitten she had just given birth to.

When I was about to have eyelid surgery, she said, I was afraid I would not be able to close my eyes again and the fear of insomnia filled my dreams. On this clear day, I cannot open my eyes and I am not afraid. Like the day my son died, the worst was behind me.

The day my son died, she says, was a normal day, but different. There were signs I had not deciphered: there were no ants on the marble counter in the kitchen, no cats in the yard, and squalls, whose long stems are the pipes through which grief rises from the depths of the earth, grew out of time.

I watch the movement of her eyelids and see her thoughts trickle down the water-covered windowpane, drop by drop, following the path marked by the first drop.

Beneath the clouds above the treetops he floats, the dead who have risen from the sand. A long trail lumbers behind him and its colour is the violet of agony. In the ultraviolet, in the black light, there is the full depth of agony.

Grains of sand fall from the dead that have risen from the sand and scratch my pupils. He comes to take my eyes, the sandman.

Then I heard the sound of thunder, the gatekeeper of the places where the living are not allowed to enter. And this is what the thunder said: Do not disturb the dead as they walk slowly on the great bridge.

I see Rembrandt looking at himself, the colour of his gaze is brown-black, the colour of the heavy earth into which he walks. When Rembrandt looks at me looking at him, his eyes are painted golden brown, the colour of compassion.

14

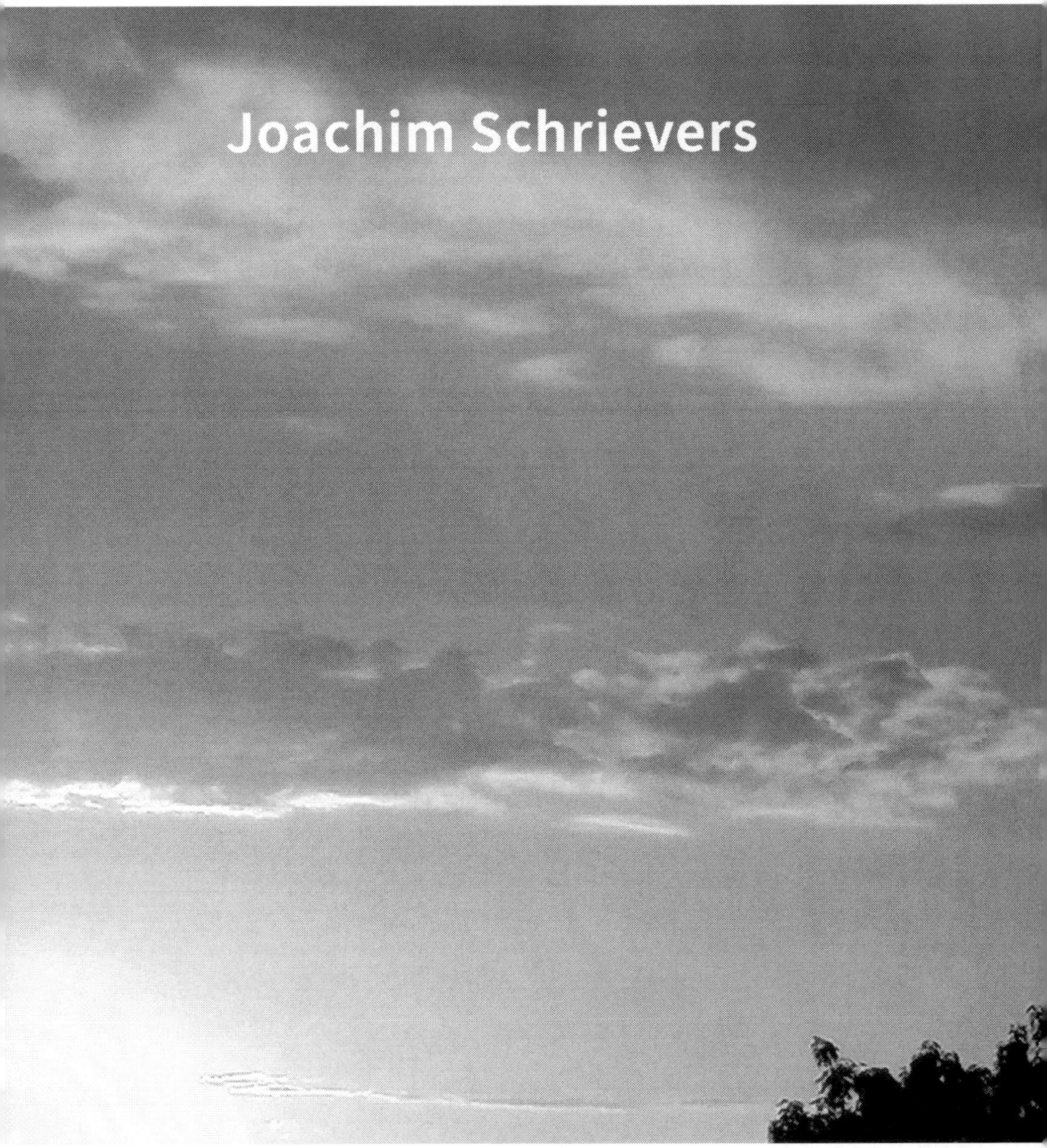

Joachim Schrievers

The Transpersonal Field of Experience as a Resonance Phenomenon

”

To experience oneself fully means to come into contact with one's inner wholeness, with the source of joy and peace. This is much more than recovery.

”

Shiatsu does help us to get well again, but first and foremost it helps us to experience that we are whole at our core.

The deep stillness and relaxation that always arises in Shiatsu opens up a space of experience for both the client and the practitioner that is markedly different from our everyday consciousness. In this space, the ill person may forget that they are ill, the weak person may no longer perceive their weakness, the dying person may forget that they have to die and the practitioner may forget their concepts.

An elderly client, who was 77 years old at the time, told me after a Shiatsu treatment that the special thing about Shiatsu for her was that during the treatment she wasn't aware of her age, which in everyday life brought about some discomfort and limitations. She felt ageless in a way for the duration of the treatment. Other clients reported having lost all sense of time and space during and immediately after the treatments, no longer feeling where their bodies began and where they ended. When asked whether this state was a pleasant or unpleasant one for them, most replied that it was heavenly and one of the most beautiful experiences they had ever had, while a few said that it was frightening as they feared losing control.

It was clear that all these people had experienced something similar, but their personal interpretations of these experiences differed significantly. One of my Qigong teachers, Prof Jiao Guorui, distinguished between so-called *small feelings*, referring to our personal feelings such as sadness, anger, fear and so on, and the *big feelings*, in which we can participate in an experience that goes beyond our personal experience, such as witnessing a sunrise in the mountains or gazing at the starry sky on a clear winter's night. The big feelings only reach us when we can, so to speak, pass through the small feelings, our personal experience, and leave them behind. Modern psychology therefore calls this *transpersonal* experience.

Such experiences have always existed in all cultures. They are inherent in us human beings as a potential that reveals to us not only a deep connection within ourselves, but also with the world around us. For religious people, these are experiences of God, more neutrally, we might call them »peak experiences«. They can leave a lasting and unforgettable impression, lead to exuberant joy, or occur so inconspicuously that our conscious selves barely notice them. They can occur in moments of self-forgetfulness in places and on occasions where they are almost expected, such as in the silence of a church, in overwhelming natural phenomena or in deep meditation. However, we can also encounter them spontaneously in situations where we think we are far away from such an experience, in deep despair because we see no way out, or in deep fear just before a life-threatening operation. People who have had near-death experiences report them, as do those who have taken part in religious rituals in various cultures. We humans seem to have both a longing for them and a fear of them.

Transpersonal experience cannot be understood, categorised or *created*. The only thing we can do is to create the conditions in which it can more easily occur. This includes experience of inner silence as well as letting go and relaxing, which leads us into a state of openness and touchability in which our resistances and fears can slowly dissipate. These preconditions are fundamentally present in Shiatsu, so it is not surprising that transpersonal experiences occur time and again. For the practitioner, these are the moments when they no longer follow the concept formed in their mind, but follow the flow of Qi during the treatment, the flow of life itself. Clinging to thoughts and concepts, no matter how coherent they may be, pushes clouds in front of the experience of one's own boundlessness in time and space. Shizuto Masunaga, my first Shiatsu teacher, recommended that at the beginning of each treatment we leave all concepts and thoughts behind and immerse ourselves in the immediate experience that opens up in Shiatsu. What we encounter then is life itself in all its dimensions.

Shiatsu is an encounter. In silence, undisturbed by everyday thoughts, client and practitioner have the opportunity to encounter themselves and each other. They do so with their respective personal characteristics, sympathies and antipathies; they encounter each other as practitioner and client in their respective roles; but they also enter a space together in which they can both put personalities and roles in order to meet anew. When space and time lose their meaning and our boundaries of space and tie blur, there is a sense of deep connection, not with the other person personally, but beyond the personal. Arthur Schopenhauer got to know this possibility of direct communication, which he described as a »fusion experience«, in the magnetic cures developed by Franz Anton Mesmer. He was so impressed by this experience that, from a philosophical point of view, he described it as the »most profound of all discoveries made«.

Franz Anton Mesmer, born in 1734, studied medicine and worked as a doctor in Vienna. Mesmer was not only an important healer (his healing successes are historically documented and undisputed), but also had the ability to induce a waking sleep state (»somnabulism«) in people during his so-called magnetic cures, in which they had access to their subconscious and could report on their dreams, visions and perceptions. These states were the precursor to hypnosis, which eventually became the basis for Sigmund Freud's research into the unconscious. Mesmer repeatedly experienced not only telepathic phenomena, but also remote effects of his treatments. He had access to a transpersonal world in which time and space were no longer limitations. Ultimately, he failed in the world of science not because of a lack of healing successes, but because he was unable to explain them in a way that was scientifically accepted at the time. Today, 250 years later, science, especially physics, is coming closer to Mesmer's experiences.

> In this new physics, there is no room for both field and matter, because the field is the only reality.
>
> *Albert Einstein*

Physicists have discovered and proven that there is an exchange of information in the universe that takes place beyond our concepts of time and space. This means that we are in contact with an information field through which we have access to knowledge that goes far beyond our personal experiences.

Franz Anton Mesmer is one of many examples of the fact that energetic medicine and transpersonal experiences are by no means a privilege of Eastern cultures; they appear wherever people turn inwards in silence. The difference between East and West, however, is that people in the East are interested in such experiences, have collected them and developed them further, whereas in Western cultures they have been rejected and fought against in the spirit of enlightenment.

When we talk about transpersonal experience, it involves a crossing of boundaries or the dissolution of boundaries. It includes the experience of oneness with things as well as with the people around you. Most practitioners are familiar with the fact that the practitioner and the client mutually influence each other through their respective energies. The vibrational fields of the practitioner and the client *resonate* with each other. The more they are on the same wavelength, the greater the resonance and thus the transmission of vibrational states. The deeper the practitioner has cultivated silence within themselves, the more deeply they can relax and let go, the more likely it is that this vibrational state will also occur in the client, provided they have the corresponding *resonance capability*.

Neurobiologist's research on mirror neurons has also confirmed in that feelings and moods can be transferred from one person to another. They now also speak of vibrational fields and resonances. Using the tools of modern brain research, they can show that when someone is in contact with an anxious person, their own anxiety centre also becomes active.

However, in the case of a transpersonal experience during treatment, it is not just a matter of exchanging personal feelings. Rather, a space of experience opens up into which both enter together and which surrounds, permeates and supports them. The more familiar the practitioner is with this space and the more secure they feel in it, the easier it will be for the client to develop the necessary trust to open up to this experience. This is because the practitioner's personal reaction to this state also tends to be transferred to the client. It is extremely valuable for the client to experience, together with his practitioner, that if they are no longer personally in control of their inner events, they are by no means out of control. In this way, the client can immediately see that there is an order that goes beyond the ego, in which life and life processes regulate themselves. In this way, the ego learns to surrender to the Self.

Again, a religious person may choose different words to describe their experience, perhaps saying that they are placing themselves in God's hands. While the experience itself is very unifying, the words and images people use to describe it afterwards can reveal differences. The experience itself is immediate and free of the personal, while the description is shaped by our biography, our faith and our upbringing. It is helpful for us practitioners to always remain focused on the experience behind the words and not to get hung up on the words our clients choose to describe it.

In addition to the spiritual dimension, such a transpersonal experience can also have medical relevance. A few years ago, I had a client in my waiting room who had tamponaded her nose. When asked why, she replied that, as usual at this time of year, she was suffering from a terrible hay fever, causing her nose to run incessantly. Alongside severe migraines, there were various other problems that she had brought up in the treatments, but not yet hay fever. I did the following exercise with her, which I had learnt in a slightly modified form from Neuro-Linguistic

Programming (NLP). I asked her to lie down in a relaxed position, close her eyes and imagine a situation in which she felt completely out of control. Once she had immersed herself in this feeling, I asked her to show me the part of her body that best corresponded to this unpleasant situation. I touched her there with my whole hand to anchor the inner image in her body. In the next step, I asked her to imagine a situation in which she felt completely at ease and in her power. Again she told me a part of her body that corresponded to this experience and again I touched her with my whole hand until the corresponding image or experience was anchored in her body. I then touched on both parts of her body with my hands and asked her to make a connection between the two touches, to allow them to merge until they were finally perceived as just one touch. She was able to follow all my instructions and felt very relieved afterwards. The next time she came to see me, she no longer had a tamponade in her nose and when I asked her how she had been, she replied that her hay fever had disappeared following the last treatment, and it remained absent for the rest of the summer. I then asked her what situations she had imagined in each case. She replied that she had first remembered a situation where she had been deeply hurt. Then she imagined the blossoming cherry tree outside her kitchen window, at the sight of which she could forget all her ailments and sorrow.

Obviously, this moment of self-forgetfulness at the sight of the blossoming cherry tree, this moment of inconspicuous peace, had an organising effect that was able to put an end to her allergic overreaction. What matters is not how intense, dramatic or spectacular the experience is, but how deeply and completely it takes hold of us. If we are not alert to such moments, we all too easily overlook them. How many blossoming cherry trees do we pass by without noticing their mystery?

This example also illustrates that it is not a matter of the practitioner's personal power being transferred, but rather that the practitioner acts as a catalyst merely making the connections to the transpersonal field of experience that is common to both and to all other people. Moreover, it shows how important the focus of our attention is, how much power can be unleashed simply by remembering an experience. In this way, a deep experience of the past can become an inexhaustible source of strength in the present. This can be experienced as a generally strengthening flow of energy or, as in the case just described, it can be used specifically to treat individual patterns of disharmony (hay fever).

The reference here to a *field of experience* is intended to express the fact that an active force emanates from this inner space of consciousness, in some ways comparable to that of a physical field, such as a magnetic field. The *Dao* of the ancient Chinese can be understood as the order inherent in life and life processes, which generates *Qi* or *Ki* as a natural organising force. Qi or Ki is the force that influences our organism as well as our psyche in accordance with this order. In Buddhism, as in Daoism, it is the »deluded ego« or the »personal body«, i. e. our personal concepts, that separate us from this cosmic order. The less we oppose the cosmic order and the forces emanating from it, the more harmoniously our lives will unfold. It is not about the fulfilment of our personal desires, but about a deep experience and letting the cosmic forces do their work.

To entrust oneself to the organising power inherent in life, in nature, to experience its workings within us, is also to participate in the miracle of nature that takes place within us moment by moment. Experiencing this creates trust, and the more our ego can let go of its fears in this process, the more this trust becomes a basic trust that is not dependent on any conditions. We cannot create basic trust in Shiatsu, and the question is whether it is even possible for us as human beings to live completely in basic trust. But it is also beyond doubt that approaching this goal in small steps of experience is great achievement.

As beautiful as all this may sound, it is nevertheless a path that is not always easy. Like most paths, it has pleasant stretches that we can enjoy wholeheartedly and rocky, steep passages that require all our strength and commitment. How we feel is not only shaped by the Self or the Dao, that supports us and in which we are always and everywhere safe, but also to a large extent by our anxious, controlling ego, which finds it difficult to surrender. The fact that a transpersonal experience can have a healing, organising effect was described using the example of the client with hay fever. However, we know from the experience of psychosomatic medicine that when our anxious and controlling ego begins to resist something, when it becomes hardened in its resistance, this can also lead to disturbances in our psychophysical balance. I have often wondered why, in the Bible, whenever people encounter an angel as a messenger of God from the spiritual world, the angel begins his message with the words: »Do not be afraid!« Obviously, even back then people knew that encounters with spiritual forces could instil fear in people. However, as we know, fear and anxiety can unbalance our autonomic nervous system and lead us into minor or major life crises. For guidance in Shiatsu, this means that the practitioner's own experience must be deep enough and sustainable enough and that they should proceed with great mindfulness.

Opening up to the realm of spiritual experiences in Shiatsu therefore also means that we may have to correct our expectations and beliefs. We can then no longer assume that every treatment will result in a feeling of well-being and improved health in the medical and psychological sense. Shiatsu is then no longer primarily a method to improve our health and inner balance, but a path to inner growth, to experiencing more wholeness and connectedness, freedom and inner peace. Ultimately, the »side effect» of this is a deeper and more sustainable inner balance, which in turn is the basis of physical and mental health. On the way there, however, it is important to say goodbye to old, previously sustainable systems and principles and to open up to the unknown, the not yet tangible.

Spiritual growth and health are not the same thing, but they are not necessarily contradictory. Illnesses and life crises always require transformation and it is not uncommon for people to emerge from them stronger and more deeply stabilised. Sometimes one might think that a growth energy driving from within was the cause of the illness rather than the bacteria and viruses found. This is especially true when a person emerges from such a process more mature and healthier.

If such inner developments are triggered by Shiatsu, the practitioner must also be available as a companion in this process. This in turn presupposes that they have travelled such a path themselves, knowing from personal experience what it feels like when the solid ground beneath one's feet slowly gives way because the ice on which one has been walking safely until then begins to melt. It is good to have solid ground under your feet, and it is good to dive into the water and surrender to this element – provided you have learnt to swim. Shiatsu can help us learn to swim, as can meditation, yoga or qigong. Here we owe a lot to the East, which has handed down to us paths travelled for thousands of years, which we can use to prepare ourselves for such experiences with a certain systematic approach.

The change that can occur in a spiritual process is similar to what a snowman experiences in the face of the strengthening spring sun. If he sees himself as a solid form, it means his death. However, if he sees himself as water that has temporarily solidified into ice, he experiences spring as a liberation in which he can return to his true nature. This becomes particularly relevant when Shiatsu is used not to improve general well-being or to correct minor disorders, but as an aid in end-of-life care, i.e. in accompanying clients through the deepest process of transformation that we humans experience. Creating an atmosphere in which it is easier for the dying person to leave their personal fears and resistance behind is perhaps the most important thing a practitioner as a companion can do.

Ultimately, however, we die many deaths in our lifetime, we have to say goodbye to people and habits. Experiencing a sense of unity and being in good hands beyond time and space helps us to allow change and come closer to our essential nature.

Life Means Being in Resonance

Whether we are happy or unhappy, whether we feel well or unwell, depends on subtle and mostly unconscious signals that the body sends and the brain receives and processes. When we are hungry, the body sends us signals that make us want to eat; when we are tired, we receive signals that tell us it is good to rest. Recognising the body's signals and following them is a natural navigation system that guides us through life. However, if we have unlearned to perceive the body's signals or have lost trust in following them, life becomes difficult because our thinking cannot replace the wisdom of the body. If you feel thirsty, you don't have to think about drinking; if you only know that you should drink, you will always forget.

But our body not only lets us feel our natural needs. It also signals dissatisfaction and discomfort, pain and inner restlessness. These signals tell us that something is wrong, that needs have been ignored and they prompt us to seek change. The body's signals are often nebulous to our mind; it is as if our body speaks a different language than our mind. And yet it seems to know something that we cannot yet grasp mentally. If we listen to the body and learn to understand its language over time, it will gradually reveal its inherent knowledge to us.

When I talk about the body here, that is actually not correct, because it is not the body, the matter, but the life pulsating through the body, the soul, from which the signals emanate. A corpse, a body abandoned by the soul, no longer sends signals. Listening to the body means, strictly speaking, listening to the soul, turning to the body means turning to the soul.

But what happens between the body or soul and our conscious self is not a one-way street. We also send signals to our body that can be helpful or disruptive, beneficial or harmful. To achieve a goal, we can demand things of our body that contradict its nature and cause lasting damage. However, we can also give it care and attention, creating an atmosphere in which it can unfold and develop freely, or more precisely, in which the soul, the life in the body, can unfold and develop freely. If body and mind are in good resonance, both will benefit from each other.

Shiatsu is a Dance with the Life Force

Shiatsu originated in a culture where body, mind and soul were never considered or treated separately, where ki, the universal life force, is equally present in language and everyday life. The Japanese term for health is genki, which is made up of »origin« and »ki«, illness is byōki, »sick ki«, weather means tenki, »sky ki«, and to be careful is expressed as ki o tsukeru, »keeping one's ki together« and the Japanese term kehai means something like »spreading one's ki (in space)«. »Man lives in the midst of ki and ki fills man« says a Chinese text from the fourth century. We do not have ki in the same way that we have muscles, bones and a body, but we are our ki. The term Ki (Qi) cannot be clearly defined. It describes a colourful world of experience (see page 170).

When our hands touch the client's back in Shiatsu, our Ki and the client's Ki begin to resonate, i.e. they begin to vibrate together. This initiates a deep exchange of energy and information in both directions. The Ki of our client speaks to our hands and the Ki in our hands speaks to our client. Ki and Ki meet and enrich each other. But the language of Ki is not the language of our mind. Most of the time, this dialogue takes place beyond our understanding. No matter how hard the mind tries to organise and understand the energetic process, it can only operate in the realm of thoughts and concepts. Systems such as the five elements, Yin and Yang and the meridians with their described functions are helpful. However, they cannot replace the experience of Ki. Only through direct experience can we grasp the unimaginable. There are musicians who have learnt to play by reading sheet music, who have studied harmony with all its facets and there are musicians who cannot read a single note and

The term Ki (Qi) cannot be clearly defined. It describes a colourful world of experience, one might even call it a world of vibration. It is described in the dictionary as

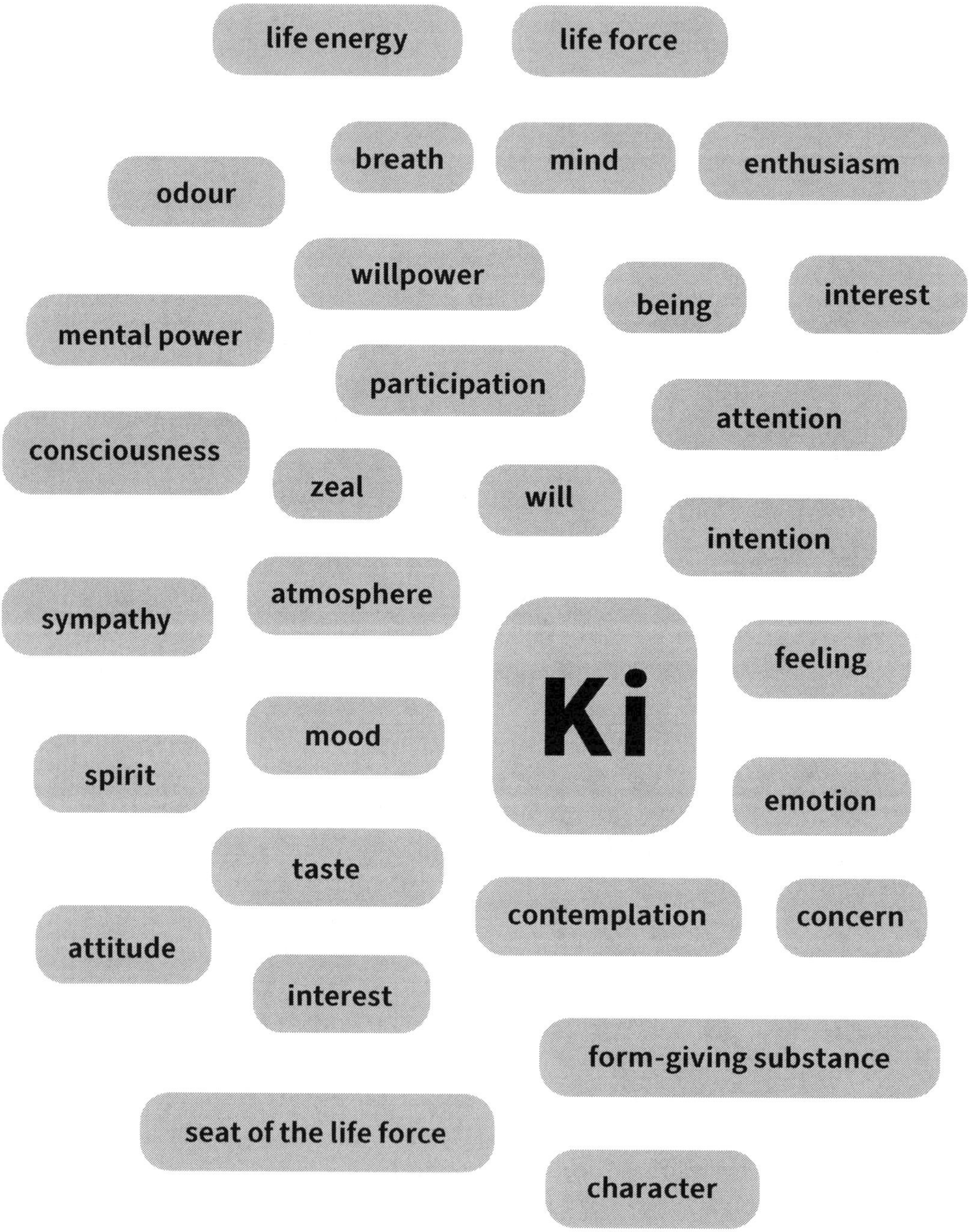

If we look up genki (healthy), we find:

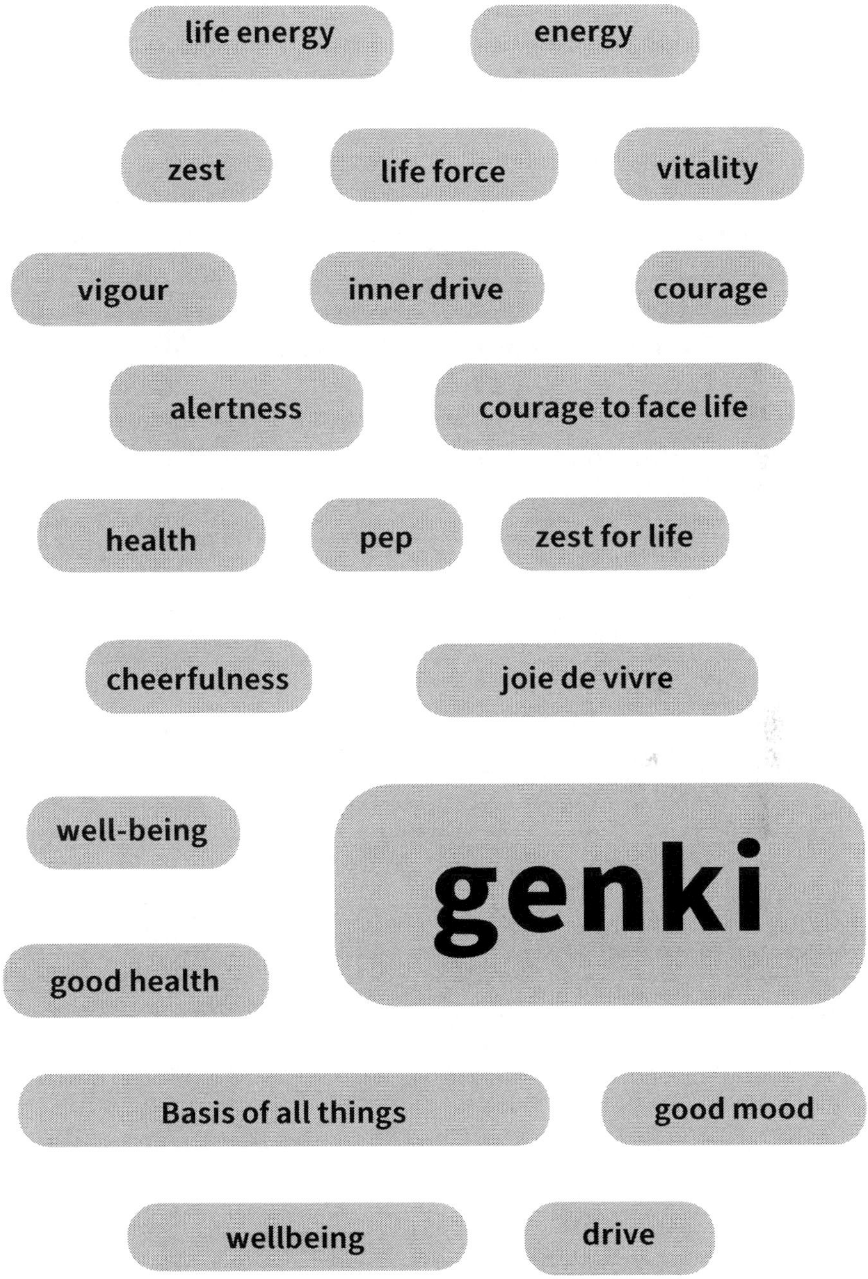

are also very limited in their technical abilities, and yet they reach people deep inside.

Shiatsu is immediate. It is an experience in which the client and the practitioner, life and the world resonate, even merge, just as the sounds of different instruments unite in a symphony. This is where life reveals itself in all its power and beauty.

Contemporary medicine is dominated by chemistry, which has researched and learnt to influence material processes down to the most subtle levels. In the medicine of the future – a hypothesis I would like propose here – physics will play a much more important role, focusing on the forces behind the material processes. It is not a question of either/or, but of both/and. All matter is nothing but energy, electromagnetic oscillation in different frequency ranges.

With our ears, we can perceive the vibrations of air molecules from 20 Hz to 20,000 Hz, which means that our eardrums can pick up and transmit mechanical waves oscillating between 20 and 20,000 times per second. Our eyes can perceive electromagnetic waves in a frequency range of 384-789 trillion vibrations per second.

But we perceive vibrations not only with our ears and eyes, but also with our whole body. We feel the electromagnetic vibrations radiated by another person through their body heat; in shiatsu, we feel the warmth of our practitioner's hands. We feel it on our stomach, back and feet, sensing how it flows deep down and changes us. Beyond the physical warmth that we can measure, we feel the warmth of the heart, that cannot be measured, and we feel the whole person touching us. We feel much more in a single touch than can be described in all the words in the world. Words describe fragments, in touch we come into contact with the whole.

To experience oneself *fully* means to come into contact with one's inner wholeness, with the source of joy and peace. This is much more than recovery. The gateway to inner wholeness can even open for the dying and make the transition easier for them. Shiatsu does help us to get well again, but first and foremost it helps us to experience that we are whole at our core.

Literature:

Bauer, Joachim (2005): *Warum ich fühle, was du fühlst.* Hoffmann und Campe.

Laszlo, Ervin (2005): *Zu Hause im Universum.* Ullstein.

Nelson, Roger (2018): *Der Welt-Geist.* Edition a.

Rosa, Hartmut (2016): *Resonanz.* Suhrkamp Verlag.

Schrievers, Joachim (2018): *Durch Berührung wachsen.* Bod Verlag.

Schrievers, Joachim (2017): *Schätze des Shiatsu.* Bod Verlag.

15

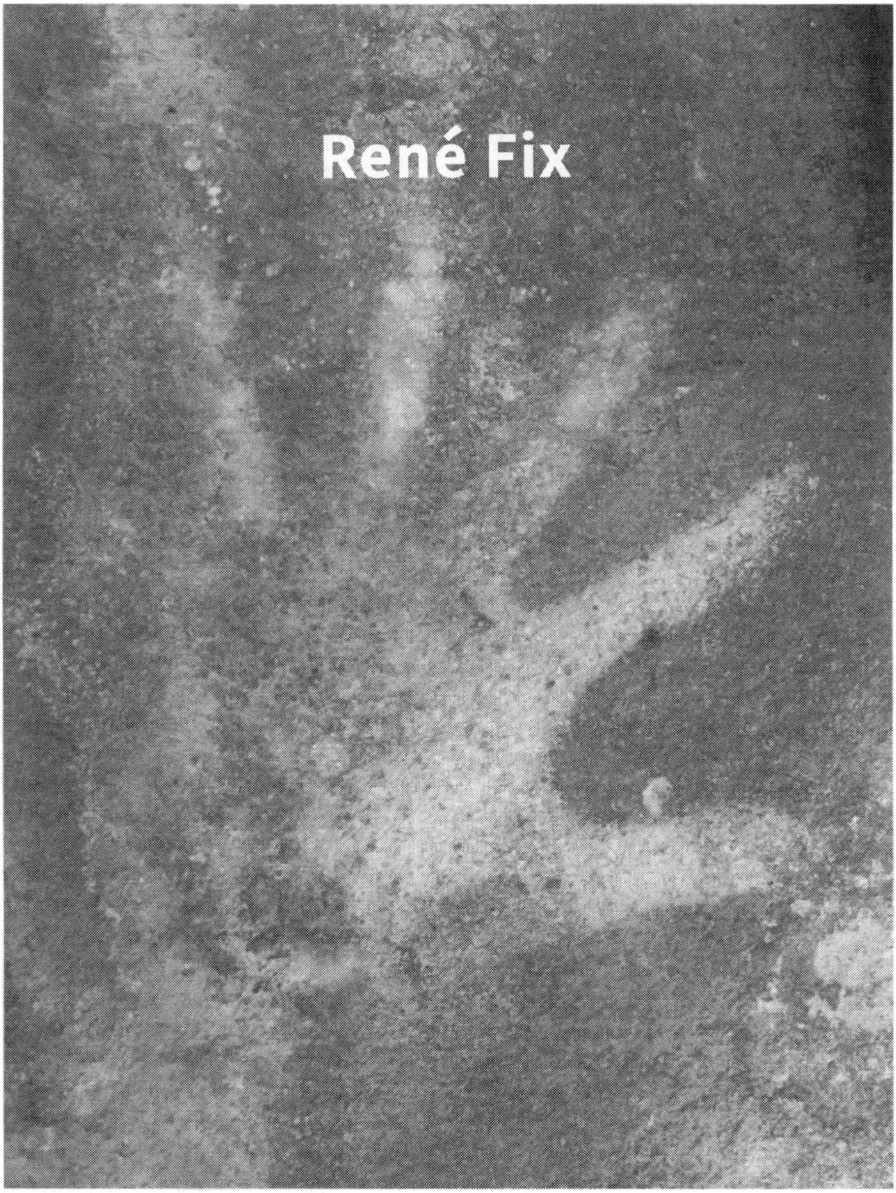

Human Dignity is Tangible

”Many years ago, I came into existence as a human being. In that creative moment when a sperm cell from my father united with an egg cell from my mother, it happened. Something new emerged from two people. And everything that comes into being has its own value. It can be named and it deserves recognition. That is dignity. It lies in the fact that something has value and that this value is recognised.

»It is what it is, says love.«

Erich Fried

I recognise myself. I am me, I want to say.
My skin, my thoughts and my identity separate me from you.
I entered this earth at a moment in the past and will leave it again at a moment in the future.
I have an opinion, an identity and a personality. That's how I experience myself.
But is that really true?
Can I be sure about it?

When I look at an apple tree with hundreds of small apple individuals, I realise that there is also a whole. The apples, the leaves, the trunk and the sap that flows through this tree form a whole, the apple tree.

The many apple trees in the orchard meadow also form a whole. The orchard is like an organism. It has its own dynamics and as this organism, it develops distinct characteristics.

The landscape made up of the meadows, forests, hills, valleys and this unique orchard meadow in turn forms a whole with its very own qualities and functions, as do the various landscapes and their inhabitants: the people, the animals and the plants. Yes, even the man-made structures such as buildings and roads together form a much larger unit – a whole, complete and yet open. It can be extended to infinity. These seemingly separate units are open to much larger units that include them, right up to the all-encompassing universe. Everything is connected. And not even that. Only separate entities can connect. But the truth is: we are as unconnected as we are unseparated. We are one.

My mind is clearly reaching its limits. After all, I can see the separation. But the truth lies beyond what I can see, smell or taste.

My five senses allow me to experience the world only at a certain level. The ancient Chinese referred to this level as »the world of 10,000 things«. Everything in three-dimensional space is defined for me at this level. This is where I feel at home as I move through this world. Understanding this level and living in it is what makes me able to act. At this level, I can sense that I am hungry, so that I can act accordingly and get something tasty to eat from the fridge. At this level, I can distinguish between good and bad so that I know what to choose. At this level, I can buy a bike so that I can get to work faster in the future.

At this level, I am in my everyday consciousness, the waking consciousness. Typically, the brain operates here with a brainwave activity of 15-38 Hz. This range of brainwave frequencies is called beta.

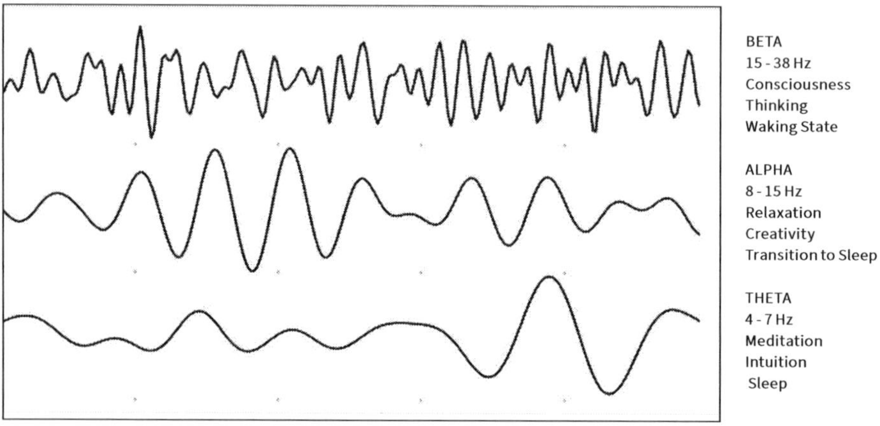

Fig.1: Brain wave activity during wakefulness, transition to sleep and sleep[1]

However, beneath this level lies a whole sea of possibilities inherent in all of us. Everyone experiences this every day at bedtime. Brain activity increasingly slows down the deeper you sink into sleep. The Identification with the 3-dimensional world diminishes and eventually dissolves completely. New information channels open up and with them new possibilities to draw from the potential of life. The potential is always there and it is unlimited, even if our thinking mind may not accept it. In order to dissolve this limitation and be able to draw from the potential, I need access to it. And in a way, I need to do it consciously. So I have to take the consciousness of the waking state with me into the opening that arises in the deep state of relaxation without falling asleep.

You can consciously slow down your brainwave activity and thus gain access to this world of potential.

For example, when we enter a deep state of relaxation (alpha) through meditation, the fixed, separate structures slowly dissolve. We become less aware of our own bodily boundaries and contact with other entities can

[1] own graphic of the author, based on https://birminghamclinicalhypnotherapy.com/brain-waves-and-trance/

occur even when there is no physical touch. New sensory and information channels open up. The five senses of sight, smell, taste, touch and hearing may still be available, but we no longer have to rely on them alone. We receive information on a different level. Everyone is familiar with this phenomenon. We often describe it as intuition or insight.

When we consciously go even deeper into meditation (theta), we no longer just feel connected to other things, we can feel directly as them. On the beta level, this seems like wild fantasising, but when we are in alpha or theta, then it is real. And it is real. We just become aware of it then.

The ancient Chinese wisdom of Taoism tells us that everything in this world is created out of the Tao:

道生一。
一生二。
二生三。三生萬物。
萬物負陰而 抱陽,
沖氣以為和。

The MEANING creates the One.
The One creates two.
Two creates three.
Three creates all things.

All things have behind them the Dark
and strive towards the Light,
and the flowing force gives them harmony.

(from Tao Te King, Lao Tzu;)

The MEANING is the Tao.
The Tao is the origin, the One from which everything emerges. In the Christianised West, we would call it God. But of course we do not mean the figurative God with the long beard. God is energy. God is without form.

God is prior to any form. Perhaps you can imagine this as a kind of energy cloud, but immaterial, just a force or a field. Now in this field direction emerges. The field is aligned in two opposite directions, The »two« are created. This polarity forms something that is given a purpose, a task. This is the »three«. Parallel to this, further directed fields emerge from this origin, i.e. further »things«, until finally everything that exists and can exist has been formed.

We can never comprehend this with our minds. We can never describe it with our language. It lies beyond that. It lies beneath everything we can comprehend. But it is there.

The TAO that can be told of is not the eternal TAO.

from Tao Te King, Lao Tzu

If everything that exists has the same origin, then this also means that this origin is inherent in everything. For that which arises from this origin does not separate itself from it at some point. Also a baby does not separate itself from its mother just because it lives outside the mother's body after birth. It remains one with its mother indefinitely. And yet this child will develop its own personality with individual characteristics at the level of 10,000 things.

The Tao is in everything. It is the lowest denominator. It is the energetic field that shapes us, anew in every moment. The field itself is infinite and without form. There is no separation. If you imagine this field as a vast smooth sea, you are a protuberance here and I am a protuberance there. In a sense, we become visible above this field. (Concepts like »above« or »below« are only tools for this image).

But if you and I are created from the same field, then we cannot be separate, or rather we are only separate if we pay no attention to the field. It is therefore a matter of perspective and thus again a matter of levels.

But let's stay with this image of the sea and the individual protuberances for a moment:

- If I move, the field (or sea) moves, and consequently, you move.
- If I think something – and thoughts are also movement – then the field moves and it changes your thoughts.

- **Everything is one.** Just as your whole body moves when you tilt your head a little to the side, everything in the world moves when you take a leap forwards.

And now it's getting interesting:
Everything is created from the field, over and over again. I am just this protuberance from the sea. A new thought does not emerge from me, from this protuberance, but it comes from the sea. From the same sea that shapes you. Everything comes from the field. Everything is the field.

- My thoughts – your thoughts – there is no such thing.
- My yawn – your yawn – there is no such thing.
- My car – your car – there is no such thing if we know about the field.

Such things exist only at the level of 10,000 things. And this level is only an excerpt of the true being.

If we accept this reality, we realise that anything is possible here. Since there are no limitations, there are also no limitations of the possibilities. Everything is possible. None of this has anything to do with our physical concept of space and time.

When you expand your consciousness to include this reality, you are forever connected to everything. And you can decide whether you want to relate to other people at the level of 10,000 things or in the consciousness of the field.

In Shiatsu, we go into a deep relaxation with those we touch. We automatically open up to the potential of the field and move away from the judgement that creates boundaries.

The pain is not bad. The leg is not broken. The soul is not crazy. Everything is as it is. Just that.

The person I work with in a Shiatsu session is, just like me, a moulded protuberance from the divine field. I meet him or her with dignity in my touch, because there is no separation that allows me to objectify this person.

The dignity of a person is what made them who they are. It is from God that this person became who they are with everything that makes them up. With all pain and suffering, with all their happiness, with their relationships, their challenges, their talents and personal qualities. And this happens continuously, over and over again. People become who they are in every moment.

Dignity lies at this interface between God and becoming. And I can touch this dignity if I free myself from the limitations of the world of 10,000 things.

To do this, we need to let ourselves in. Shiatsu makes this letting in possible. I don't think in terms of body structures. The material is something I can refer to, but it is only one phenomenon of life. In Shiatsu, I touch life itself. I open myself up to the magic of life and let it guide me. It is always happening now. Now I enter into an encounter. I immerse myself in this miracle and encounter the deep primal force that shapes life, in the material as well as the immaterial. The person »speaks« to me and lets me know what they need to make change possible. Because it is always about change. Life is about unfolding. Just as every flower unfolds moment by moment to reach its full size and eventually wither and die, so individual human life continually develops within us. There is an ongoing process of becoming.

This becoming arises from the primal force of the Tao. Ki (Qi, breath of life, energy) flows through the human being.

Shiatsu is the art of communicating with this Ki and accompanying the process of becoming.

16

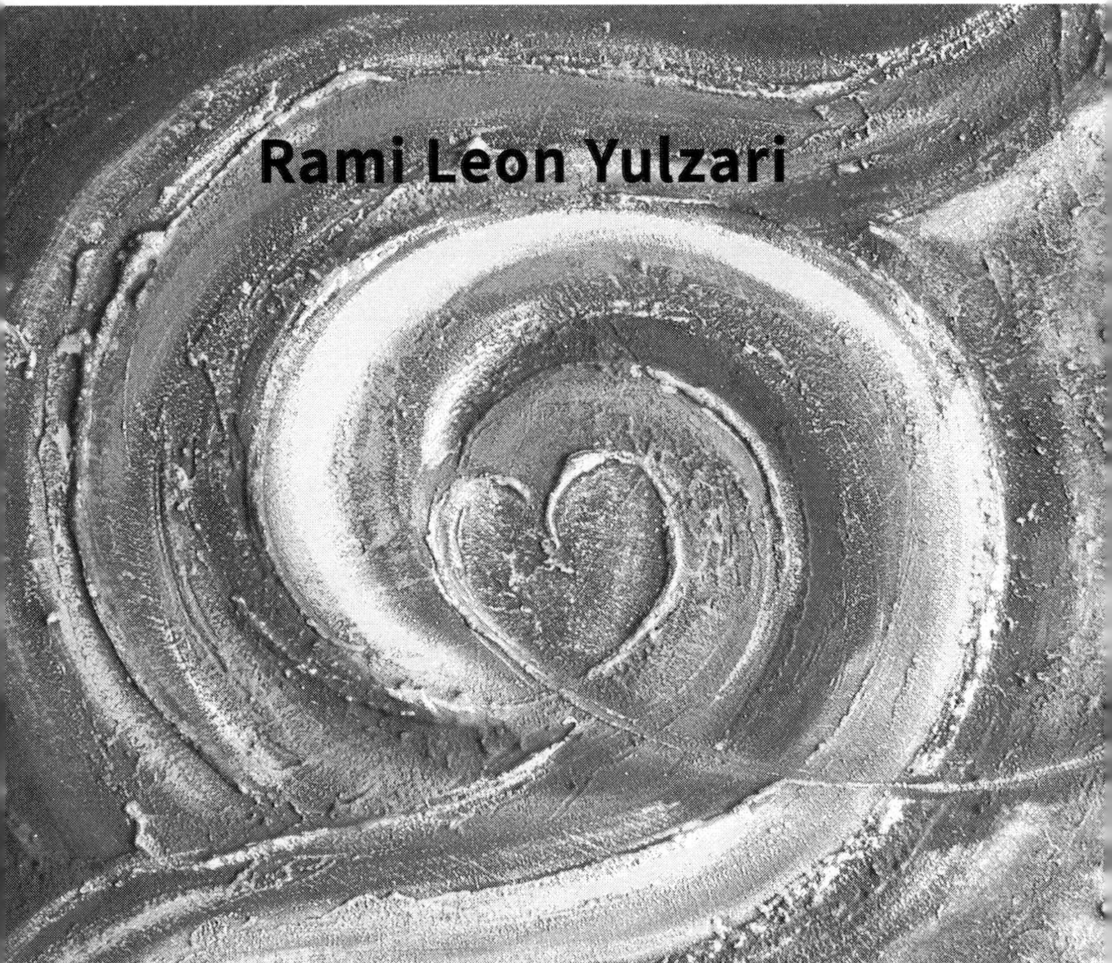

Sound of the heart,
now!

” The quality of a Shiatsu treatment
is maternal and
its heart
is supportive.

To the mothers –
Hanna, mother of Hagar and Nitzan
Hagar, mother of Reef and Lyle

THE CODE

»Without memory and without desire« is how the psychoanalyst Wilfred Bion instructs a therapist to meet a patient. In »Notes on Memory and Desire«, Bion says: »Psychoanalysis is not looking at what happened and what will happen, but what happens«. These words simply say: no past and no future, a continuing present. They also encode a secret, a message that has not yet been deciphered.

I am looking for a code, a signpost. Maybe they are words in the phonetic alphabet, like echo-bravo. Maybe these words are random code names, like wolf-meeting. Sometimes these words are clear, they do not hide, and yet they are incomprehensible, like fire on our forces, and you wonder who is afraid there, who has been wounded there, who has died there, and whose grandmother will weep. I remember the funeral of Mony, it took several months before they found his body in the sands of Sinai. I heard his grandmother weeping over his grave in Ladino, and I thought how rude it is to change the order of the world, to bend the course of time, a grandmother weeping over the grave of her grandson. On the other hand, if time is just a continuous present, it is possible to call him: Mony, Mony do you hear, over, your grandmother is crying for you, over, the world orders have changed and the course of time is reversed. You can come back, over and out.

Time and duration

Tsutomu Oshima is the »Shihan«, the chief instructor and founder of the »Shotokan Karate Do« association. Oshima is one of the greatest karate practitioners and teachers of our time, if not the greatest. I saw a video of him saying: »The old masters knew how to stop time«, and he demonstrated: one of the senior student attacked him with a very fast fist. Behind that speed we can find decades of training, a very great speed. There is no doubt that an untrained person would not see the blow coming and approaching him. Even an experienced karate practitioner would find it difficult to react to such an attack. Oshima moved slowly against the attack, a slowness that struck me as laziness, anticipating the attacker for a relatively long time and deflecting the fist with embarrassing ease. Like an adult playing with a child who is trying very hard to win, but in no way can.

It seemed that when Oshima spoke of stopping time, he was referring to a significant slowing of time. In his demonstration, he showed his ability to see the movement of the attack before it came towards him, while it was still intended. This gave him a lot of reaction time, the ability to react at a chosen moment. The gap between the speed of the attack and the speed of the defence was so great that the explanation of slowing down time does not seem sufficient. Oshima seemed to move at a different time, which can be described as follows: two people are standing in front of us, facing each other. One is training to increase his speed relative to time, while the other is moving at a different time; Oshima and his student are moving as if they were at different times. Oshima called it »stopping time« and he was actually demonstrating his ability, probably the ability of the old masters, to be in another time and from there to meet the time we are used to. As if they could go in and out of the flow of time at will, as if it were a not particularly strong stream of water, a dip in a spring, rather than the usual image of a brutal struggle with the sweeping, checkered flow of life.

The idea of two times and the image of time as a stream of water recalls the philosopher Henri Bergson's idea of Duration. Bergson distinguishes between scientific time, »logical time«, which is measurable time – hours, days, years – and time, which he calls »Pure Duration«. The real, original time, according to Bergson, is fluid – flowing, mobile, constantly changing. Linear time, the product of our minds, makes the fluidity of time disappear. In his book *The Creative Evaluation*, he writes:

> »If everything is in time, then everything changes inwardly, and the same concrete reality never recurs. What is repeated is some aspect that our senses and especially our intellect, have singled out from reality, just because our action, upon which all the effort of our intellect is directed, can move only among repetitions. Thus, concentrated on that which repeats, solely preoccupied in welding the same to the same, intellect turns away from the vision of time. It dislikes what is fluid, and solidifies everything it touches. **We do not think real time.** But we live it, because life transcends intellect.«

The source of our knowledge of Duration and our ability to continue our connection with »life transcending intellect« is experience.

The experience of floating on water, when our eyes are closed and we surrender to the rhythm of the waves, and at the same time we are in an inner reality; the feeling of drowsiness before falling asleep; when our body temperature rises and we hallucinate; when we take off in a plane into the clouds, experiencing the feeling of being separated from them and after a while becoming airy like them, moving with any random breeze, gusts generated by changes in atmospheric pressure that we cannot perceive with our senses. We experience floating in-between, an experience that has no time, where we lose our physical reality and our pain, and maybe we stay there forever. We feel the other time, time that is not measured, that has no beginning and no end.

In these experiences the laws are different, as W. G. Sebald describes in his book *Austerlitz*:

> »It is not the time that is controlling the lives of people but the weather, which means a dimension that cannot be quantified, a dimension that the linear uniformity is foreign to, that does not move regularly forward but moves round and round under the influence of accumulation and outbreaks, and comes and goes each time in a different way and do not know where it is heading.«

Weather is all present time. To be present is to be in Duration, in what has no direction and moves in circles, to experience chance in every moment and often to experience chaos without creation.

At the beginning of time

Let us look at early postnatal life. Here they are, a mother and a newborn baby. The mother is lying, still heavy, with the baby on her chest, his eyes closed. She looks at him with a small, exhausted smile on her face. The experience of pregnancy and birth is still with her. When she raises her eyes, her gaze seems dreamy, far away. A thin net is spread over the mother and child, separating them from their surroundings. It seems transparent. It is impossible to pass through it. They are in their own world, in their own time.

The psychoanalyst Donald Winnicott describes the relationship between a mother and her newborn as a unit, »the mother-baby unit«, inseparable, two »live an experience together«. In the first period of his life, the baby is totally dependent on his mother. The mother is required to give herself completely to his needs in an absolute match. Winnicott calls this match »Primary Maternal Preoccupation«. In his book *True Self, False Self* he writes:

> »(...) Towards the end of the pregnancy and for a few weeks after the birth of the child, the mother is preoccupied with the care of her baby, which at first seems like a part of herself: moreover she is very much identified with the baby and knows quite well what the baby is feeling like. For this she uses her experiences as a baby. In this way, natural provision is made in nature for what the infant needs which is a high degree of adaptation«.

In this way they experience a break with the normal course of time. All the processes of a living infant constitute a »going-on-being«, that is, being in a continuous present.

The mother continues to hold her baby in a kind of womb after the birth. She wraps her baby and herself in a thick blanket, and they both breathe the warm air underneath, which is their common breath. This image gives the impression of defence; the mother is protecting the baby with her body from any suffering and from time lurking outside. She rejects time from the outside until her baby's total dependence is transformed into relative dependence with the child's growing autonomy.

I suggest that we see this particular time as a memory of what Bergson called »real time«, which we forget as we move away from it as we grow. Winnicott implies this. The mother, he says, remembers and uses her experiences as a baby.

The psychoanalyst Thomas Ogden, in his book *On Not Being Able to Dream*, develops Winnicott's idea and argues that in this first period of the baby's life, time is perceived as a threat. The mother's role is to protect the baby from time. The measured and fixed time threatens the baby's survival and therefore protection is required, which in turn requires sacrifice and devotion on the part of the mother.

> »The main function of the early psychological and physical holding, involves isolating the baby from the unchangeable, unrelenting otherness of time. When I talk about the otherness of time, I refer to the experience of the baby of »time made by humans«: time of clocks and calendar, of day and night and so on. Time in all these forms is a human invention (even the concept of day and night) and has nothing to do with the experience of the baby ... in fact, the earliest holding of the mother includes

> her entrance to the baby's sense of time, thereby creating the illusion of a world where time is measured almost entirely in terms of the physical and psychological rhythms of the baby. These rhythms include the rhythms he needs for sleep and wakefulness, contact with others and isolation, the rhythms of hunger and satiation, the rhythms of breathing and heartbeat.«

In those early weeks, Ogden says, the mother absorbs the impact of time on her baby by giving up her own needs, her own separate time. Our experience, I would argue, is different. When we look at a mother and her newborn, we experience a special serenity, an extraordinary softness and a sense of surrender without concession. We get a clear feeling that wants to go on and never stop. The mother-baby experience is one of a lifetime, and the outside world is usually a disturbance, a disturbance of the hammock swing, a noise that violates the unusual silence. To return to the inner rhythm is to return to Duration, to real time, and the time of the clock is the illusion in which we all live.

Being in Duration is being with ourselves, with our most inner rhythms, this is our ability to act in the world from deep listening to ourselves.

Health and illness

The peculiar condition of the mother after birth is called by Winnicott »illness«. It is an illness that can only develop when the mother is healthy. It lasts for a few weeks after birth and then disappears and is forgotten.

> »Mothers do not remember it easily after they have recovered from it, and what they do remember they tend to repress,« says Winnicott. »A woman must be healthy to develop this condition (»almost sick«) and to recover from it when the baby releases her.«

I suggest that we see the »illness«, our ability to be in Duration, as our health. We are healthy when the ability to move between time and Duration is available and effortless. In other words, we do not experience a struggle between times, which is a struggle between our inner and outer world, between our inner and outer rhythms. The inability to hold the possibility of Duration creates a collision between the outer and inner rhythms, a conflict that affects our health.

The healthy mother connects with the Duration of the baby, which becomes her Duration, which is the memory of the time after her own birth. The ability to enter and exit the flow of time into Duration is probably the ability given to mothers and probably to the Ancient Masters, as Oshima thinks. We can therefore see the Ancient Masters as Ancient Mothers rather than Ancient Ancestors.

We know that the ability to step out of the flow of time is essential to our health. We know this because if we do not fulfil this need, it is forced upon us, we are ill. Sebald describes it this way in *Austerlitz*:

> »... Being out of time still exists even in the city of London, the Metropolitan of time. After all, the dead are out of time, and the dying, and the many patients lying in their own homes or in hospitals. And not only them, after all, one portion of personal disaster is enough to disconnect us from any past and from any future.«

The sick, the wounded and the dying, the weakest among us, are isolated in areas where reddening windows signal sunset, the voices of nurses changing shifts mark the end of night and the beginning of early morning, and the sound of instruments, some deep, gloomy and slow, others beeping, thin and frequent, separate time inside from time outside. The time outside makes the people outside forget the rustle of the time inside, which is the rustle of life and death.

This is being that is not Duration. This is a detachment from regular time, a detachment that turns pain into suffering.

Pain and suffering

The philosopher Emmanuel Levinas, in his book *Time and the Other*, describes the experience of insomnia as that which makes us aware of our separation from time.

> »This time is not an imaginary experience. Insomnia is constituted by the awareness that it will never end – that is, that there is no longer any possibility of withdrawing from the vigilance to which one is held. Vigilance without end. From the moment one is riveted there, one loses any notion of a starting or ending point.. Here, time begins nowhere, nothing moves away or shades off ... Vigilance without possible recourse to sleep.«

The experience of insomnia, according to Levinas, is an experience of distress, of suffocation, of hopelessness, it has no space, no time and no end.

As in the poem *Lullaby* by the poet Sharon Hass:

> »... the man awake in the late hours of the night, the late hours when at the bottom of every staircase another staircase opens and the hole grows«.

I make a distinction between pain, whose time is limited, and suffering, which is pain whose time has stopped, whose duration we do not know, and above all whose end we do not know. The mother reassures her child who has fallen and injured himself by saying that the pain will soon go away. She is relaxed and confident that it will, and the child in pain discovers after a short time that in fact the pain has passed and he forgets about it. He learns to distinguish between pain by its quality and the time it takes to recover. The doctor diagnoses that the flu will be over in a week, and so it is. By following the mother, the doctor and learning from the experiences of others, the child can tell when the pain will go away. Pain that does not pass in time, that remains, that becomes chronic, that has no end in sight, becomes suffering. The sufferer's life revolves around the pain in a kind of endless circle, without direction or purpose; it largely dictates his lifestyle, his attitude to himself and to his surroundings.

Over time, the suffering becomes more intense. The pain that has stopped and turned into suffering continues to refer to the fixed time. The sufferer is left behind and sees with longing eyes that time goes on without him.

Pain is in measured time. Our dialogue with pain allows us to recognize its diversity, each of which carries a message. The one who feels pain can limit its duration, either by himself, by his experience, or with the help of others, by their experience.

Pain becomes suffering when the rhythm of time is lost, when we do not see its end. When the possibility that it will never end, or even increase, becomes a real and only possibility, accompanied by fear.

In suffering, says Levinas, loneliness is revealed in all its cruelty: no one or nothing can help. Suffering is a convergence within myself, so that nothing can separate me from myself. The sufferer collapses inwards without choice, imprisoned within himself. He falls into a deep, dark hole and all he can see is the further fall, deeper into a darker place.

The therapist reaches out to the patient, brings down a rope and sometimes descends into the hole, the bottom of which is not visible. There, holding hands, they wait for the moment when the patient can look up and see the light that marks the exit, and then begin to climb up.

Being with the patient in his loneliness is the therapist's way of bringing him back to measured time. The sufferer who can see the possibility of the end of his suffering in time, his suffering becomes pain and pain becomes bearable. From there the therapist will lead his patient into the warm bosom of Duration.

Duration of Shiatsu

The Shiatsu patient lies on a mattress on the floor, with his or her weight gravitating downwards. His or her outward movement has stopped almost completely. What is visible now are spontaneous movements – the movement of the pupils under the eyelids, the corners of the mouth, vibrations in the fingers, an inner growling voice, a sudden jump in the leg or the pelvis, intestinal sounds, odours from inside the body finding their way out.

The therapist's hand rests heavy and soft, sinking into the patient's body. Ripples are created around it, expressing the patient's internal rhythms that respond to touch. The therapist's hands fumble for a match. They sink down like into wet sand on the seashore. Wide and large, they spread into the patient, becoming part of the vibration that is his life. The ripples spread out from the touching hand and return to it like an echo in the mountains, going back and forth. This is the movement of life in which the therapist participates for a moment. He experiences the loss of a sense of time, which is his attachment to Duration. His feelings and thoughts rise to the surface and sink again like a bird gliding on an invisible breeze, gliding in a dream.

The Shiatsu therapist slows down his movement. He listens to his inner movement and allows it to respond to the movement he encounters on the outside. He pays attention to the gap between the patient's outer and inner movements and tries to bring them closer together. He suspends. Being in suspension allows for change. What seems chronic, repetitive, can be different. Being in suspension is the possibility of connecting with Duration, and what seems to be slowing down is being in another time.

In a supportive and containing Shiatsu therapy, the patient returns to their inner rhythm and the ability to connect with it. As he becomes more connected to the experience of Duration, he will find his place, his center, his home. Following Winnicott, we can emphasize the maternal quality of Shiatsu treatment, that its heart is support. Winnicott's »mother-baby« unit is not a preparation for the world and the future, but the connection between the inside and the outside that we strive for in our adult lives as we negotiate with external time. Throughout our lives we are constantly trying to bridge the gap between our inner rhythm and our ability to listen to and connect with it, and what is outside of us.

The quality of a Shiatsu treatment is maternal and its heart is supportive.

Following the Chinese spirit, we can say that it is a connection to the earth quality. The therapist gives the patient the earth to rest on, gathers him and connects him to the heavy movement of the earth moving on its axis. The therapist connects with the movement of the patient's energy, the rhythm of inhalation and exhalation. He responds to changes in the movement, accompanying and supporting it, like a mother cradling a baby in her hands, in the rhythm of the heartbeat. The therapist and patient now listen together to the sound of the heart.

Duration of Qigong

The Qigong practitioner stands. He has practiced standing for many years so that his weight falls down without resistance; he lets go and does not hinder gravity. The center of his body, the pelvis, is very heavy. His legs are like growing roots. At the same time, his torso is drawn up, the top of his head is connected to the sky, light, effortless. His shoulders are loose, his arms hang from them, his neck is open, his chin is tucked in and he looks forward, far into the horizon.

The beginning of the movement is outwards. The practitioner practices a series of movements, trying to be precise. The outer movement becomes slow, circular, does not stop and has no effort, its rhythm is steady. An inner echo of the movement is created. After a long period of training, the external movement becomes instinctive. The form is done by itself, without thinking and without effort, by listening to the inner movement. Then inner and outer movement become one. Sri Nisargadatta Mharaj says in his book *I Am That:*

> »Going out is natural in the beginning and
> going in is natural in the end,
> but in reality the two are one,
> just as inhaling and exhaling are one«

The qigong practitioner is standing. His movement is very slow. He is silently examining the boundary between movement and non-movement. He is still. He is examining the boundary between stillness and silence. He is moving from movement to stillness, silently. He is very awake without alertness and without reaction. He experiences lightness and heaviness together. His attention moves easily and quietly between his feelings, his emotions and his thoughts. He is not paying attention to anything, he is dreaming and waking at the same time. He is experiencing Duration and from there he looks at time.

Heart sound, now

The Qigong practitioner pays attention to his inner time; the shiatsu therapist pays attention to his inner time and the inner time of his patient. They are attentive to the time outside of time, between life and death. The ancient Chinese who practiced Qigong thought that through training they would transcend death. They believed that by achieving a balance between inner and outer movement, and between themselves and the mysterious movement of the universe, they could stop the time that leads to death. In this way they become one with nature and become immortal or gods, but not human beings, whose humanity lies in their death and their choice between movement in time, which they have created, and being in Duration.

Shiatsu therapists and Qigong practitioners stay between movement and non-movement, listening to the sound of a string just before it stops vibrating, or perhaps the sound before it is created, which is being in Duration. Staying in Duration allows one to pay attention, to listen more and more delicately to an original sound, a primordial vibration somewhere within, without words. There we are, as T.S. Eliot describes in Four Quartets: »… like a Chinese jar still moving in its stillness«.

And in the silence we listen to the sound of the heart, now.

Literature

Bion, Wilfried (2017): *Notes on Memory and Desire.* In: Wilfred Bion: *The Los Angeles Seminars and Supervision*. Carmel Publishing, S. 214.

Bergson, Henry (1974): *Creative Evolution.* Magnes Publishing, S. 123.

Hass, Sharon: *Lullaby.* In: Haaretz Newspaper, 21.09.2016 (Übersetzung ins Deutsche von B. Murakami).

Levinas, Emmanuel (2014): *Le Temps et L'autre.* Hakibbutz Hameuchad Publishing, S. 20f.

Ogden, Thomas H. (2011): *On Not Being Able to Dream.* Am Oved Publishing, S. 258f.

Sebald, W. G. (2006): *Austerlitz.* Keter Books, S. 87.

Winicott, Donald W. (2010): *True Self, False Self.* Am Oved Publishing, S. 280f.

17

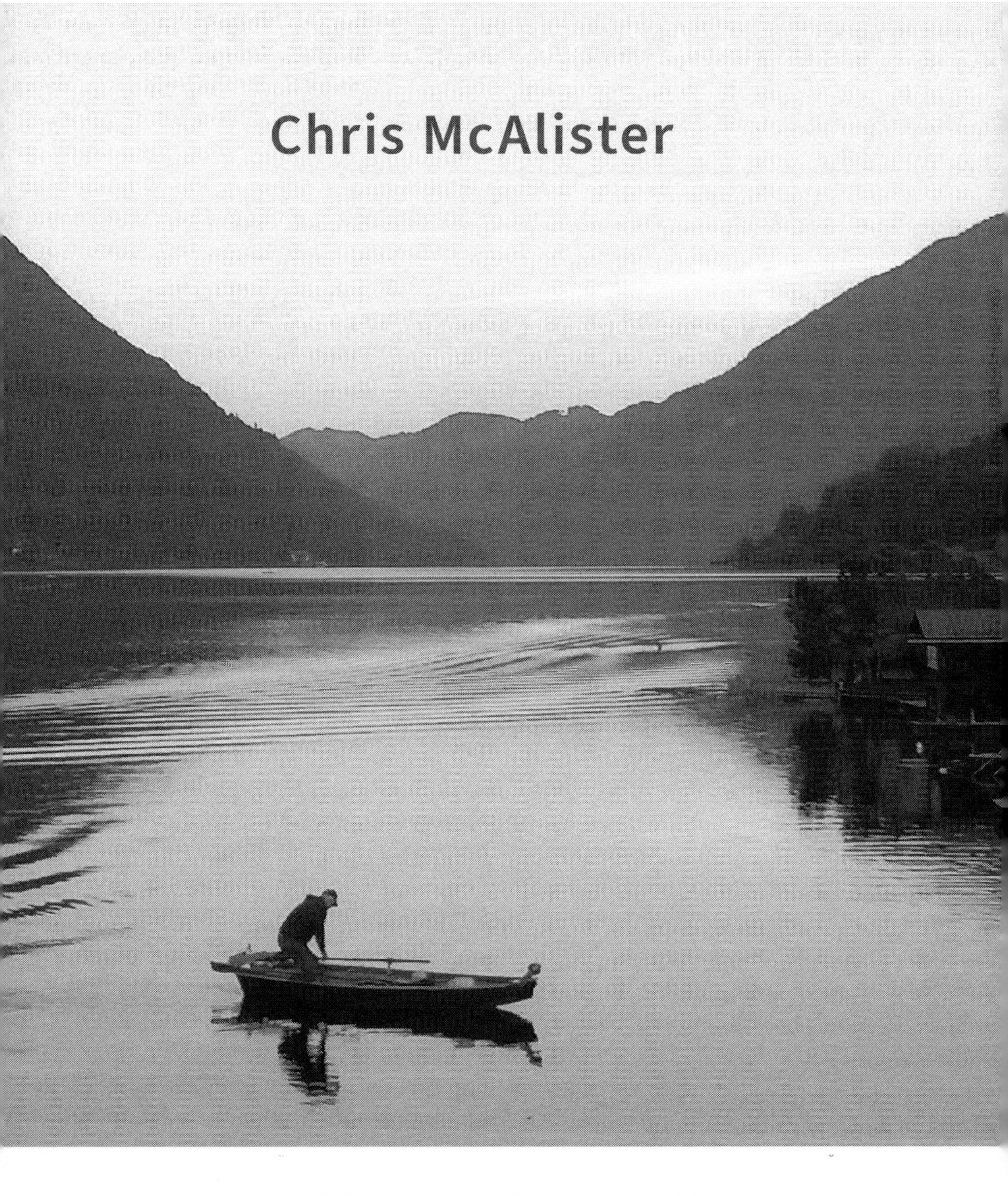

Walking the Talk

When
we study Shiatsu, we allow it to seep into our skin, our movements and finally our very consciousness.

When
we practice Shiatsu, it gradually becomes part of our way of look-ing at the world. The more we live with Shiatsu, the more we become Shiatsu in our everyday dealings.

When
we teach the principles and techniques of Shiatsu, we allow them to determine the choices we make and the decisions we take.

Shiatsu has been in existence for around 100 years. It has been here in the West for around half of that time. Some feel that things are going too slowly, and that Shiatsu has not made the breakthrough into the hearts and minds of the common man that it ought to have done by now.

We look at the enormous benefits we have received on our way to becoming practitioners, we observe the effects of the treatments we give, we revel in the multi-level transformations we regularly witness among our clientele and we wonder: why don't more people want this? How come we are not begged to appear on morning TV shows, radio programmes and web podcasts all over the world every day to tell people of the miracle in our hands?

How can it be that Reiki is on its way to becoming a household name? Why is massage and even Thai massage the stuff of everyday conversations but not Shiatsu? How come acupuncture is routinely discussed (albeit with plenty of skepticism) but Shiatsu still hides in the shadows?

There are probably very good partial answers to all of these questions and some of them lie completely beyond our power to affect in any way. We cannot alter the fact that acupuncture has been around for thousands of years and is attractive to medical personnel and naturopaths in a way that Shiatsu never will be. We cannot alter the fact that millions go on holiday to Thailand and receive treatments – an inexpensive session in the local high street massage parlour is obviously a lovely way to bring back holiday remembrances. This is an advantage Shiatsu will probably never come close to having.

Another pertinent question: how is it that students have been falling away from Shiatsu in recent years? Shouldn't they be coming to our schools in droves to partake of our special and arcane knowledge? Well, let's do the math very swiftly. Thai massage training can be done for a fraction of the price and in a very short space of time. The same applies to massage. Reiki can be »mastered« in a matter of months if you have the financial muscle. Shiatsu takes three years. Realistically and conservatively speaking, if you want an authentic Shiatsu diploma from a reputable school, it takes three years or more – and that is exactly the way we have decided we want it.

We have striven to set up what we believe are realistically high standards for Shiatsu training in every country and even on a European basis. In fact, one might argue that the standards are not nearly high enough. In the European arena, efforts are fairly well on the way now to formally establishing the profession of Shiatsu and the training levels we will have to insist on will, almost certainly, be substantially higher than they are today. The argument goes roughly as follows: once we have a real profession, we can insist that the required level of training truly reflects the professional status we yearn for and claim to deserve. We will be able to call the shots and schools will be full of people lining up to take their place in a profession that can stand straight-backed and tall.

We are not quite there yet, however, so the discussion remains an interesting and fertile one. What will it take to make Shiatsu a household name?

The work going on in National associations and the European Shiatsu Federation has been in progress for thirty years or more. It is slowly but surely showing signs of bearing fruit in the foreseeable future. In the meantime, what can be done at the other end of the spectrum – the grass roots, if we might use that term.

Each and every student, practitioner and teacher of Shiatsu has a valuable role to play in this regard. Some are less interested than others and that is perfectly fine. Not everyone wants Shiatsu to become a household name and that is a reasonable opinion to hold. Many prefer to stay under the radar, off-grid and out of the limelight. There are excellent reasons for this, and no arguments are necessary around that topic.

But for those of us who would like to see Shiatsu – finally – take its place as a profession among others, what might be the best way to proceed? I believe the answer may be as simple as it is undramatic: walk the talk.

If you love doing Shiatsu, be Shiatsu. If you enjoy being part of Shiatsu classes, gatherings and teachings, become Shiatsu with your person as well. If you practice Shiatsu as part of your livelihood, make sure it becomes part of your lifestyle as well. If you teach Shiatsu, make sure your life becomes a lesson in the applied principles of Shiatsu. If you run a school, be sure to run your life in the same way – holistically and according to the ideas that form the basis of all we do in our lessons and course plans.

A central question then becomes: What is Shiatsu?

There are a million responses to this and once we've looked at them all, a million new versions will mutate forth. We will never be able to exhaust the question because it is one that is subject to change and fluctuation, just as the principles underlying it prescribe: change is the only constant. We know this from day one of our Shiatsu studies when our teacher showed us the Yin-Yang diagram, the Taiji Tu. The moment the flow between polarities stops is the moment of death. We fervently hope that Shiatsu will not die and therefore we accept that we will never be able to capture its true essence more than fleetingly in words or concepts: the Dao that can be described in words is not, and never will be, the true Dao.

How then to define this wonderful, ever-changing, multi-faceted art we love so much? If we cannot define it, then obviously we have to allow each other to describe it in different terms and to include and exclude different features. No two people will be able to agree on all aspects of what is or is not Shiatsu. For the sake of appearances, in the various political arenas and when dealing with the »outside world« we coin descriptions and decide on definitions. We hope that they will not appear too contradictory from one school and organisation to another, but differences do exist and will continue to do so. We have to learn to live with this, for it will always be so. It will continue to be so simply because each individual approaching and experiencing Shiatsu does so in a unique way, every single time – a living miracle that we all celebrate on a daily basis.

Returning therefore to the main question under consideration:

How to walk the talk when we cannot agree on the language?

It is clearly not easy to discuss this in any definitive way. Principles are all we have, and freedom is something we all rightly insist on.

When we study Shiatsu, we allow it to seep into our skin, our movements and finally our very consciousness.

When we practice Shiatsu, it gradually becomes part of our way of looking at the world. The more we live with Shiatsu, the more we become Shiatsu in our everyday dealings.

When we teach the principles and techniques of Shiatsu, we allow them to determine the choices we make and the decisions we take.

Some people prefer a quiet and solitary approach – they welcome their clients into the space they have created and work in an individual and in a sense perhaps »pure« fashion. Others combine it with other methods, blending techniques from other disciplines and creating hybrids.

Some work in close collaboration with other therapists from completely separate modalities, hoping in this way to combine the best of many worlds in a symbiosis that benefits the »client in the centre«.

Still others have the firm intention of taking Shiatsu into the mainstream via pain clinics, maternity wards, elderly homes and hospices, even prisons and remand homes.

There is literally no end to the number of possibilities of working with Shiatsu and walking our talk.

The more time we spend with Shiatsu, the more we become Shiatsu. Perhaps, ultimately, this is the only way Shiatsu will become a part of everyday life. Let's continue to walk the talk and patiently allow Shiatsu to seep into the movements, thoughts and awareness of those around us. It may not happen fast; it may proceed like a glacier, almost imperceptibly and maybe that's a good thing.

The movement will persist as long as we persevere.

AUTHORS

René Fix

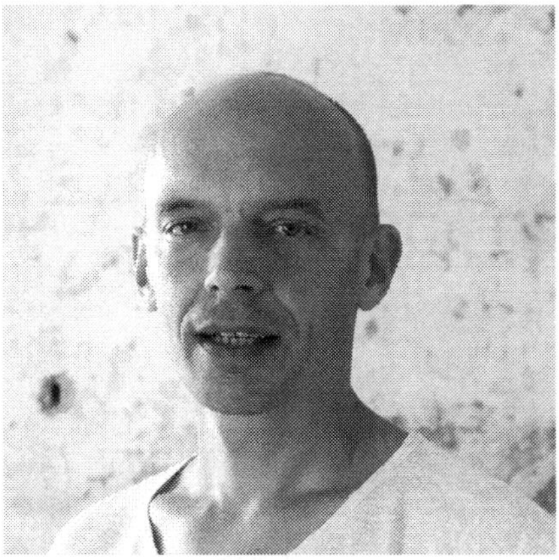

René's great curiosity about the movements of life and his passionate interest in nature have been with him since childhood. After studying forestry, this led him to work as a forest mapper, which allowed him to spend a lot of time in nature and experience it up close.

Shiatsu came into his life in 2004 and was expanded and deepened through many training courses. In 2016, René took over the European Shiatsu Institute in Heidelberg, where he himself had completed his training. A new field and a new potential opened up. Today, this school is called kiCollege, stands on completely new foundations and pursues a new path of learning and growth with a very open concept. René's great curiosity about the movements of life and his passionate interest in nature have remained with him since childhood. After studying forestry, this led him to work as a forest mapper, which enabled him to spend a lot of time in nature and experience it up close.

Contact: renefix@posteo.de

Heidy van Koesveld

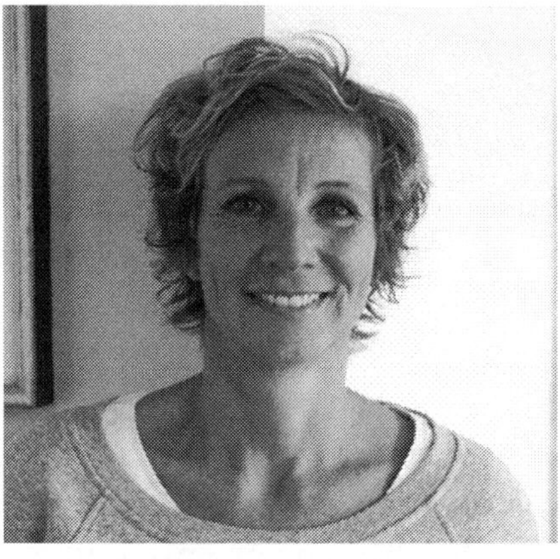

Heidy began practising Shiatsu in 2009. A student of Joyce Vlaarkamp, she runs a practice as well as teaching at the Zen Shiatsu School in Amsterdam. She was actively involved in the organisation of the International Shiatsu Congress in Amsterdam 2020. "She says about the focus of her work: „The quality of contact during shiatsu is something that inspires me and at the same time sparks my curiosity. This in itself can be a lifelong study.

Contact: heidy@studioki.nl

Chris McAlister

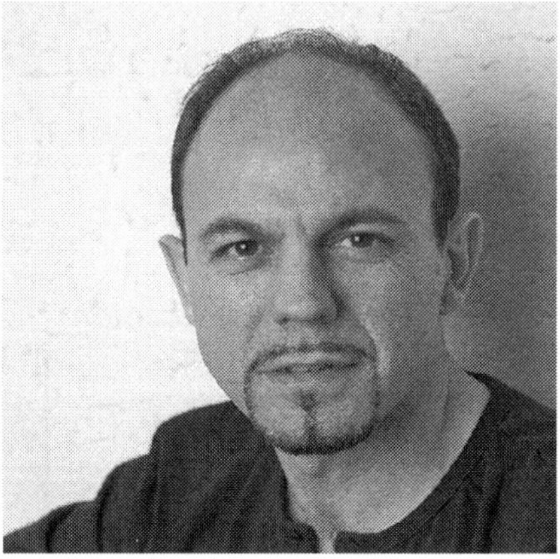

Chris encountered Oriental medicine while extremely sick in East Asia in 1986. Sessions with practitioners from Tibetan, Ayurvedic, Homeopathic and finally Chinese medicine showed him the immediate and long-term benefits of traditional, holistic practices.
He began his formal Shiatsu studies in the UK, studying at two different schools simultaneously, and continued during a five year stay in Japan with Takeo Suzuki, a close student of Masunaga's final years.
He is currently President of the ESF, the European Shiatsu Federation.
Contact: chris.mcalister360@gmail.com

Barbara Murakami

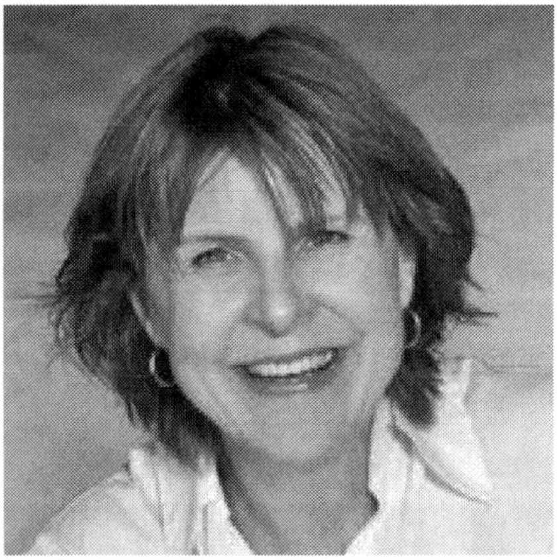

In her day job, Barbara Murakami worked for 40 years as a special school teacher for children with behavioural problems. She has been a Shiatsu practitioner since 1997 and a Shiatsu teacher since 2007. In 2008, she completed training in psychosynthesis, which is a form of psychotherapy based on depth psychology. The experience gained from this and from numerous other further training courses in Focusing, Clean Language, Seiki and Qigong are incorporated into her shiatsu, working with Qi in its various forms at body and mind levels. Shiatsu with difficult children and adults with severe multiple disabilities in particular has opened her eyes to what Shiatsu is essentially about: meeting and being with what is.
Contact: barbara.murakami@gmx.de

Bill Palmer

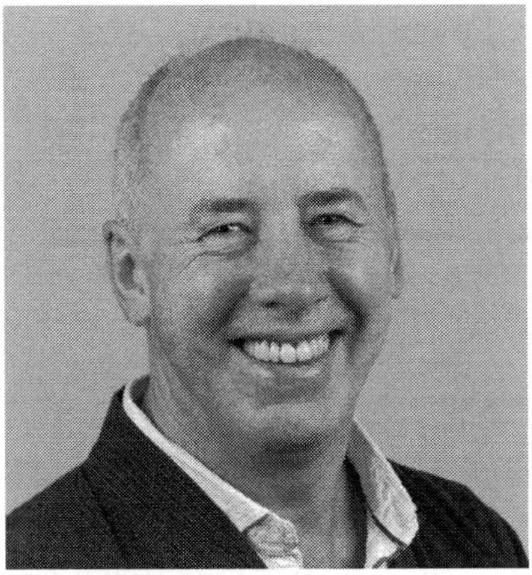

Bill Palmer is the Director of the School for Experiential Education and has been studying Shiatsu since 1973. He was one of the pioneers of Shiatsu in Europe and created and edited the Journal of Shiatsu and Oriental Body Therapy. He is the originator of Movement Shiatsu, a highly interactive form of Shiatsu, focused on helping people to be aware of themselves through the body which he teaches worldwide with his wife Teresa Hadland.

Contact: bill@seed.org.

Nick Pole

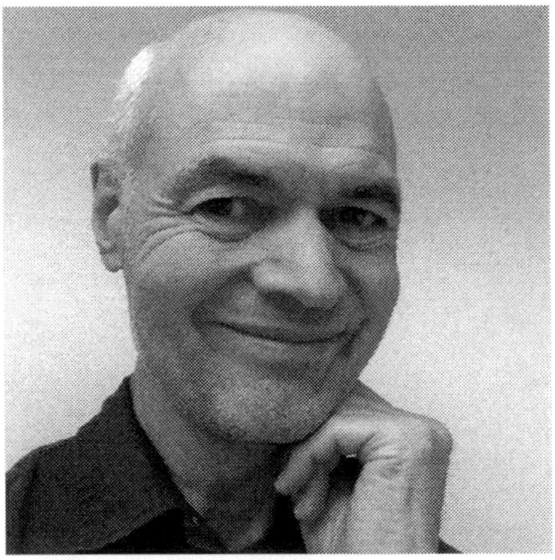

Nick Pole integrates language, mindfulness and bodywork into his work. Nick studied history and political science and then worked as a film-maker for 10 years. Following an illness, he discovered acupuncture and shortly afterwards began studying Shiatsu at the Shiatsu College in London. He has been teaching Shiatsu since 1992. He also trained in NLP and in Seiki with Akinobu Kishi. Whilst trying to integrate the different approaches he came across Clean Language, a wonderfully simple and effective way of helping clients to listen to themselves in a deep, body-centred and authentic way. He has written a book about it and is increasingly incorporating Clean Language into his teaching. He has also been teaching Mindfulness Based Cognitive Therapy since 2012.

Contact: nickpole33@gmail.com

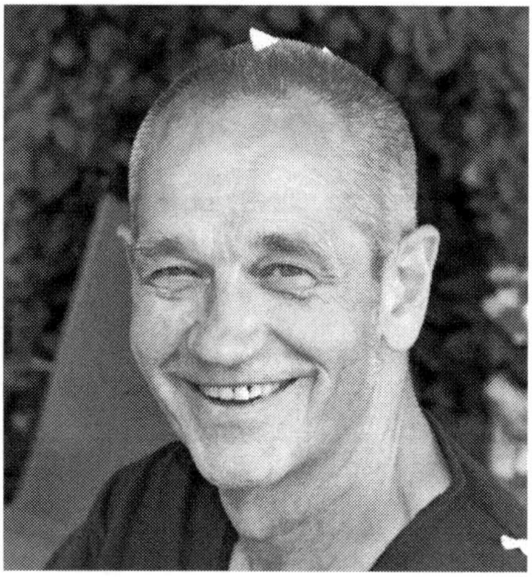

Wilfried Rappenecker

GP, founder and for 30 years director of the School for Shiatsu Hamburg, Germany. For many years director of the International School of Shiatsu (ISS) Kiental, and the European Shiatsu Conferences Kiental, Switzerland. He is co-founder of the Shiatsu Society Germany (GSD) and author, co-author or editor of seven books on Shiatsu as well as numerous articles.

Contact: W.Rappenecker@fuer-shiatsu.de

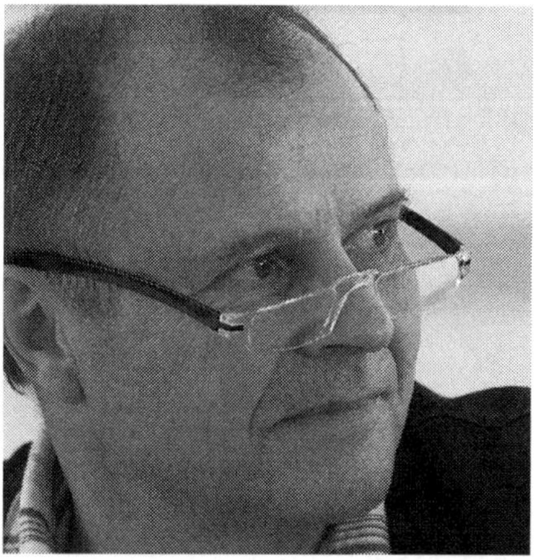

Joachim Schrievers

After studying sports science at the Cologne Sports University, he became interested in Zen meditation and the connections between body and mind, movement and consciousness. During a two-year research scholarship at the Tokyo Sports University, he learnt Shiatsu from Shizuto Masunaga, Taiji from Yang Ming Shi and practised Zen with Yamada Kōun Rōshi, and later with his successor, Kōun-An Rōshi. In the early 1990s, he studied Qigong with Prof Jiao Guorui.

Meditation, Qigong and Shiatsu are the foundations of his energetic work, in which he has been combining and practising Eastern wisdom and Western knowledge for over 40 years.

Contact: ek@schrievers.net

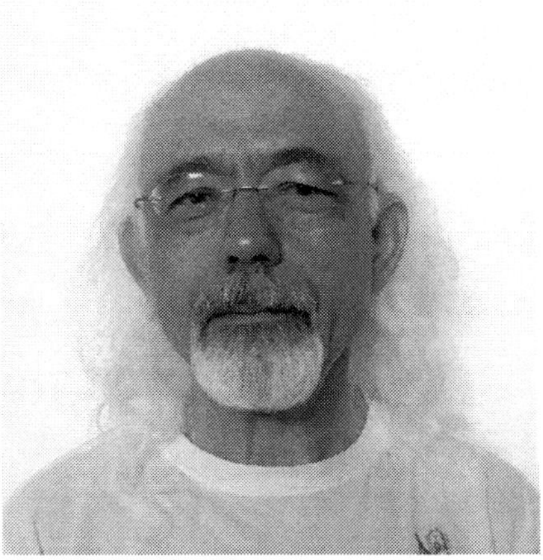

Rami Leon Yulzari

Rami practices and teaches Shiatsu and Qigong in Israel and Germany. He is the former director of »Maga« School of Shiatsu in Jerusalem.
In his practice and teaching, he emphasises qualities of touch and movement: Paying »Gentle Attention« to inner Qi and the way it meets outside Qi, through touch and movement.
He is inspired by Zen-Buddhism, Psychoanalytical thinking, Art in general and literature and poetry in particular.
Contact: ramiyulzari@gmail.com